The Thinking Person's Guide To Permanent Weight Loss

JON PERLOW

THE TWINING PRESS, MILL VALLEY, CALIFORNIA

Cataloging Information

Perlow, Jon
    The Thinking Person's Guide to Permanent Weight Loss

    1. Reducing.   2. Reducing—Diets.
3. Reducing—Psychological Aspects.   4. Weight Control.
I. Title.
RM222.2P475 1986   613.25   85-52342
ISBN O-936877-02-2

Cover design by Michael Hollyfield, Sonoma, California

Manufactured in the United States of America

This book is lovingly dedicated to Marjorie Perlow, my mother, from whom I inherited my sweet tooth and from whom I also received limitless love and lots of good advice.

Acknowledgement

My most sincere thanks to Dr. Allan Wolfe, Bronni Galin, M.F.C.C., Faith Sale and Mary Jane Schramm whose comments on the manuscript were invaluable in helping me sharpen the focus of a number of my thoughts; and to Kathleen Flanagan, a very special lady who typed the manuscript; offered much valuable feedback on the clarity of the prose; and tried her best to overcome my resistance to following some of the rules of writing the English language, which in the interests of communicating more clearly, I manage to disregard.

Contents

Why I know what I am talking about.

The valuable lessons that I learned in giving up cigarettes which helped me get my weight, and will help you get your weight, under control.

In this chapter we begin to get into the swing of things; we start to direct our minds appropriately; set our focus and our mood; then take our first important step along the path to effective, enjoyable weight control.

Short definitions of two terms that I made up in order to help get certain points across.

Now we are into the heart of the matter. This chapter will get you thinking in a new way about the problem of weight control; seeing things in a way that will enable you to deal with it successfully. Even if you don't buy this book, read this chapter.

How to solve the problem discussed in Chapter 5 and thereby set yourself on the path of freedom from the torments of overweight forever.

A. Low calorie foods that you can consume in almost limit-less quantities and not gain weight.
B. An example of substituting lower calorie meals and snacks for higher calorie ones without any sacrifice in satisfaction.
C. The number of calories a person uses in doing popular recreational athletic activities.

A listing of the number of calories in just about anything that you eat. This guide is unique in that it not only gives the number of calories contained in a particular portion size, as do all calorie guides, but it also gives the number of calories contained in an ounce of the food. This additional information makes it possible to easily ascertain the number of calories in any size portion, not just the portion size described in the guide (which in the real world is almost never the size of the portion we eat).

Caution

Before you undertake any weight control program that is intended to result in a substantial loss of weight; and which can involve changes in your daily diet and/or in the amount or strenuousness of the exercise you do, you should consult your doctor, to see if he or she has any advice, suggestions, or cautions to offer. "An ounce of prevention is worth a pound of cure."

Foreword

If you have ever been on a diet and lost weight, you can lose weight again. If you have ever lost weight, you can keep it off. The secret is simply to be in the right frame of mind. That's what this book is all about. Getting you into and keeping you in the right frame of mind. Getting you to effortlessly and enjoyably switch your addiction for food to an addiction for responsible weight control. I did that; so can you!

Despite thousands of books, many by respected physicians and other professionals, despite a proliferation of reputable organizations helping people to lose weight, despite an increasing amount of low calorie packaged foods, the proportion of the nation that is overweight today is not substantially different from the percentage of the population that was overweight thirty years ago, when I went on my first diet. The fact of the matter is that diets, diet clubs, and diet books are only support mechanisms. They are useless to a person who is not in the right frame of mind and truly unnecessary for one who is. This book will show you that weight control is about learning a skill, not going on a diet. Effortless, effective weight control is a simple skill, but one that nonetheless must be learned. This book will teach you the skill and put you into and keep you in the frame of mind to effortlessly use this skill.

Certain of my experiences have really made a difference in my frame of mind. What these experiences had in common was that they changed the way I understood something. That's what this book is designed to do: to cause you to think about things in a new way, a way that will make a difference, a way that will allow you to enjoyably and effectively get your weight under control, as I finally have. I keep my weight steady, right where the life insurance charts say it should be for a person my height and body frame; seventy-five pounds less than I weighed when I began the last diet I will ever have to go on.

Even if you have to lose a hundred pounds or more, what I say will work for you. Even if it seems so long, so hard, so impossible, even if you have tried and failed many times. And on the other hand, this book is also for you if you have but a few pounds to lose and feel, "I don't need him," "I'm not addicted to food the way he was," "He's talking to someone else." Know that if you are constantly having to lose five pounds or more, and you are always struggling, worrying about losing those few pounds, I'm talking to you. Keeping it off is really what this book is all about. Taking it off only lasts for a few weeks or months. Keeping it off lasts a lifetime.

[1]

About Me

THERE ARE TWO THINGS that you need to do, to once and for all, effectively and enjoyably control your weight:

**ALWAYS EAT WHEN YOU ARE HUNGRY
READ THIS BOOK**

After you read this book, I think you will see how controlling your weight can be simple, interesting, stimulating, and satisfying.

Let me begin by asking a crucial question: Why is it that although millions of intelligent, reasonable people know that if they weighed less, they would feel better, look better and live longer, and that when they overeat, they feel physically and/or emotionally distressed—why is it that these intelligent people don't do the reasonable thing which is to lose weight and keep it off? My answer to that question will surprise you, and it is really understanding the answer that sets one on the path to freedom forever from the torments of overweight. By the way, the answer has nothing to do with liking food too much, having no willpower, or being emotionally upset, answers that might come to mind initially. But before I answer this big question, let me tell you a little about myself and my way of doing things.

I am a fellow sufferer. Not a theoretician, dietician or doctor with a new fad diet. I have been in the trenches. I've been on more diets than I could possibly remember. So many that I often refer to myself as the leading lay authority on the diet. Through the years, I have lost the best part of a ton. And I didn't go on namby-pamby diets. A diet had to be worthy. My goal was usually to lose at least fifty pounds over a period of many months. Just to make the game interesting, I once quit smoking and went on one of these gargantuan diets at the same time. I had been smoking six packs a day. (You see, I don't do things in a small way.) I did quit smoking and did lose a lot of weight. I never smoked again. That was nine years ago. But alas, the weight came back and there were more diets. In all fairness, I should tell you that I had once before quit smoking for five years, and had started again because I became very angry at my former wife. Talk about self-destructiveness! Well, I have learned a lot since those days that has enabled me to understand my addictions and how to get rid of them without pain.

Not only do I dislike pain, I abhor discomfort. I spent six months in basic training in the Marines, including three months at the notorious Parris Island, and I never spent one night sleeping outdoors. That was quite a trick! I used another trick to stop smoking cigarettes, though at the time I did not really understand what I was doing. (I'll tell you how I stopped smoking in the next chapter, because it taught me certain things that would later help me to get my weight under control.)

I also used to drink fifteen to twenty cups of black coffee a day. Maybe thirty years or so after the first cup (it takes me a while to catch on), I began really noticing the effect the coffee was having on my physiology. I would feel hot; frequently perspire; I would be charged up; my heart would be racing a bit. Then, four years ago, I was at a biofeedback seminar and the leader, to illustrate a point, described how the caffeine in coffee went to work directly on the involuntary nervous system something like a shot of adrenalin would. The understanding that I was giving myself something akin to fifteen to twenty shots of adrenalin a day confirmed what I was noticing about the way I felt after drinking coffee, and I didn't like it. I walked out of the workshop and decided to give up coffee. I haven't had a cup since.

I quit smoking because it hurt so much. The first time (for five years) I stopped after walking up three flights of stairs at a YMCA, following a game of squash with a friend. I wasn't in very good shape to begin with, and this fact plus the cigarettes (then only three packs a day) really made me hurt. The pain got to me and I quit. Later on, the second time around, when I was up to six packs, it hurt to laugh, cough (which I was doing a lot of) or even walk at more than a crawl. So again, the pain impelled me to stop. Just as with the black coffee, I didn't like the way I felt and I was worried about my health.

Well, the same was true with eating too much. I didn't feel good, and I knew that it wasn't good for my health to be overweight. (Not to mention that my body looked so lousy that I had to keep it hidden under bulky, baggy clothes.) With cigarettes and coffee, I could quit cold turkey. Never had another cup of the black stuff or one of those foul-smelling weeds again. Eventually, the craving weakens, and finally, finally, finally dies completely. If you stay off the stuff long enough, not only don't you crave it any more, you start to find it offensive. But that takes a long time. For years I would still enjoy smelling smoke in the air at the office, in a restaurant or other public place. But now it makes me so uncomfortable that I have to leave a room in which there is a lot of smoke. To a lesser extent, I also find the smell of coffee offensive.

However, with food, there is a difference. And it is a big difference. You can't quit cold turkey. One has to eat to live. And therein lies a great danger, because eating often feeds on itself. As an old potato chip ad used to say, "You can't stop after eating just one." Further, food is invariably an accompaniment to our celebrations, and it is a primary way we socialize with other people. Through meetings, parties, coffee breaks, get-togethers, and teas, a lot of our everyday activities are associated with food; food that is often made particularly tempting, and usually particularly fattening. The fact that one can't banish food completely from one's life intensifies the danger of relapsing into overeating, which is an addiction just as cigarettes, alcohol, and black coffee are addictions. However, once one truly understands the problem and how to deal with it, the danger will become less and less. Finally, it will not be possible to overeat. It will hurt too much. You won't be able to overeat unless you are so self-destructive that you are willing to endure enormous pain and discomfort. And understanding the problem and how to deal with it successfully and painlessly is really very simple.

[2]

How I Stopped Smoking

ONE SUMMER when I was in college I traveled by car across the United States with a friend who wanted to give up smoking cigarettes. He bought a book on how to stop smoking and while I was driving, he read a few pages aloud to me. I don't remember the name of the book or anything my friend read to me except the sense of the first line, which went something like this, "Relax! Light up a cigarette! Don't worry! Take it easy! Go ahead, enjoy the cigarette!"

I don't remember how much of the book my friend read, and I know he smoked for at least another ten years, but that opening line has stayed with me and come to influence my way of handling my addictions. Minimize the unpleasantness. Limit the feeling of threat. And make the job as easy as possible.

The title of this chapter could as easily be, "How I Got a Lot of Attention," as "How I Stopped Smoking," because the method that I used so successfully to give up smoking got me a lot of stares and caused a lot of comment. In fact, although I don't normally like attracting attention to myself, I may have prolonged using this little artifice long after it was necessary to do so, because I secretly enjoyed the ado I was causing. I could have stopped after a few months. In reality, I continued for a few years.

What I did was to first buy a pack of cigarettes. I opened

the pack and put it in my pocket as I always had. Then when I felt the need for a cigarette (which, as I had been smoking six packs a day, was almost always at first), I would take one out of the pack and put it in my mouth where I would let it dangle unlit. From time to time, I would hold it in my hand and put it in an ashtray as I would have done with a lit cigarette. When the tension was really great, I would eventually bite off and immediately discard the filter and dangle the rest of the cigarette from my lip. Little by little, I would bite the cigarette down to a smaller size, discarding each bitten-off piece. The cigarette kept vanishing just as if it had been puffed up in smoke, though it usually took considerably longer to disappear. Finally, I would discard the remnant of the cigarette and, at first, go right to the next one. I went from smoking six packs a day to, at first, dangling and chomping to bits one and a half packs a day.

I came to realize that when you walk around with an unlit cigarette dangling from your lip which you occasionally bite on, discarding the chomped-off piece into an ashtray or other receptacle, you are doing something a little bit out of the ordinary. People tend to notice things that are out of the ordinary. Especially if you happen to be dangling the unlit cigarette in such places as a No Smoking section of a restaurant or a store, in a theater, or in an airplane prior to takeoff. People would constantly be telling me that I couldn't smoke in this place or that. I used to get so much attention from the stewardesses on airplanes prior to the plane taking off; first telling me that I couldn't smoke and then, after realizing the cigarette wasn't lit, talking to me about what I was doing; that a male business associate who flew with me a few times said that he might take up the habit. Once a little old man who had obviously been propelled by his wife to get up the courage to do so, came over to where I was sitting in the No Smoking section of a plane, leaned over and told me this was a No Smoking section. I pointed out to him very gently, as I always did, that the cigarette in my mouth wasn't lit. A little abashed, he struggled back to his seat and I heard his wife ask in a very eager, loud, whispering voice, "What did he say?" The man responded, "He said it wasn't lit." "Oh," she sort of moaned. For a moment I was sorry that the cigarette hadn't been lit, so I could have given them the satisfaction of putting it out.

During the years I was dangling cigarettes, I went to work for a company as part of a new management team. A co-worker who had been with the company before I arrived and with whom I later became friendly, told me of how the existing employees would, as could be expected, discuss, describe, and assess the new managers. She said when I was first described to her, all anyone said was, "He chews cigarettes." She said she couldn't believe it. Who could?

Many people reject my method of giving up cigarettes either because they don't want to attract attention and/or they think it doesn't look good and/or they think it's messy (which it really isn't when compared to scattering ashes and leaving stubs or larger pieces of smoked cigarettes all about). I don't really like attracting attention (at least I don't think I do). I don't like doing things that don't look good. And I don't like being messy. However, I did want to give up smoking cigarettes, and this method made it a lot easier for me to do so. Thus my first lesson from this experience was that if you really want to do something badly enough, and you find something that works for you, disregard any minor social consequences that may arise.

The real lesson, though, that I learned from giving up smoking in this manner is what it taught me about dealing with an addiction. The easiest way to give up an addiction is to give up as little as possible and satisfy as much of the needs surrounding the addiction as one can without giving in to the addiction. By having the cigarette available, I knew that if I really, really, desperately needed one, it was there. I was safe! By putting one in my mouth when I felt the urge for a cigarette, I was satisfying my oral need to have something in my mouth, which was very much part of the gratification I got from smoking. By taking the cigarette out of my mouth frequently and holding it in my hand, or resting it in an ashtray, I was satisfying a need to do something with my hands, which was an expression of inner tension. The taste of the tobacco, which I could experience after I bit the filter off the cigarette, enhanced the experience. When I really needed a drag, I chomped down on the cigarette and to some extent this chomping action would help relieve the inner urge I was then feeling for the smoke to come pouring into my lungs.

I soon discovered that there were very few occasions I really, viscerally, internally craved the feeling of smoke in my lungs. Almost always after a cup of coffee at the end of a meal, and in moments of very high tension, I would feel my body looking for the relief that it could get from the inhaling of smoke. But almost all of the other times that I was dangling the cigarette and fiddling with it, I was satisfying some urge other than the one the inhaled smoke was needed to subdue. I estimate that well over 90 percent of the time I was smoking cigarettes, I didn't need to actually smoke them to get the type of gratification they were providing. Thus I realized that to help get rid of an addiction, one has to understand what it is that one is craving and give oneself as much as one can of that satisfaction without also feeding the addiction. Carrying this idea over to the area of dealing with an eating addiction, I realized that one must never be hungry. One simply needs to learn in a nonfattening manner to satisfy the needs for *stuffing* and *good tastes* which are the two things that cause people to overeat.

Another important thing I learned about addictions from giving up smoking, is that addictions really do fade out. They go away. They go away so completely that after a while, the addictive substance can become unpleasant. While it may be true that some substances may be a lot easier for certain people to become addicted to, it is also generally true that we become addicted to what we are used to. Our bodies are extremely adaptive. Stop doing something and the urge to do it will fade away in time. As I said earlier, today I am offended by the smell of smoke. I must leave a room when it becomes at all smoky. It is really true that that to which you attract yourself becomes familiar and addictive. Thus, all other things being equal, if you stop eating hot fudge sundaes and start eating apples, you can be sure that in time (possibly not in the few weeks or months that it may take to lose ten, twenty or fifty pounds, possibly a lot longer), you will stop wanting hot fudge sundaes and will prefer apples. Knowing this can make it a bit easier to eat apples (or other low calorie foods that you enjoy) instead of hot fudge sundaes if your goal is to take off weight and keep it off.

There is one thing about my method of giving up smoking that many people think would make it impossible for them to use it. They feel they would yield to the temptation of lighting and smoking that cigarette constantly dangling in their mouths. They are sure they would succumb. Maybe! But if you really want to give up smoking, before you prejudge the method, try it. If you have the *intention* not to smoke, you are not going to light up a cigarette. (In the chapter on intention, you will see that intention not willpower makes things happen automatically.) Once you have the intention not to smoke, putting the cigarette in your mouth is an aid in actualizing that intention. If you first put the cigarette in your mouth, expecting the cigarette to do it for you, it won't. You have to not smoke it, or smoke it. The cigarette won't do that on its own. But the unlit cigarette being in your mouth can make it easier for you not to have to light up because it will be giving you so much of the satisfaction that a lit cigarette would also be giving.

Everything starts with really meaning to make it happen. Not waiting to see if it really will happen. Once you really intend to stop smoking, or to control your weight, then knowing how to help yourself out by dangling a cigarette and chomping down on it, or eating something when you are hungry, will make it a lot easier to maintain the intention and turn the intention into reality.

[3]

Knowledge Is Power

THIS BOOK EXPLAINS certain basic principles of weight control as I have come to understand them. This book is not about dieting, psychology, or behavior modification, though ideas from these fields are involved in understanding weight control, and I do talk at times in terms that are associated with these subjects. But when you understand basic concepts of weight control, diets, behavior patterns and psychological states of mind, all become irrelevant considerations. We are dealing with a very simple subject. Weight control really boils down to what you are going to do at the *critical moment* when you realize you are hungry and have the urge to eat something. You can only do one of three things: (1) don't eat and become increasingly uncomfortable; (2) eat something and subdue the urge; (3) try to make the urge go away. Those are the only possible solutions to the problem of what you can do when you are hungry. And that is the point of our focus. Put in a less didactic form, the problem is: *"Now that I'm hungry, what am I going to do?"*

There are two ways to deal with any difficult problem such as how to once and for all break the gain weight-diet-gain weight-diet cycle. One can either struggle, or one can, as the Buddhists say, use skillful means to overcome the problem. Skillful means might best be illustrated by the art of jujitsu, where effort is minimized and size advantages are overcome by using leverage to turn the momentum of one's opponent against him or herself. Struggle doesn't need to be explained. It's hard, unpleasant, and most often unnecessary—certainly so when it comes to losing weight. In my view, doing things the easy way is by far preferable to struggle except in a few isolated instances when struggle may be good for you, such as when you are trying to build up muscles by doing pushups, deep knee bends, and other strengthening exercises.

For many, many years and many, many diets, I had essentially been struggling to lose weight. And from what I can see, almost everybody else who is dealing with their weight is choosing the way of struggle. It was not until I learned how to stop struggling and start using skillful means that I truly became successful in controlling my weight.

What I am going to do in this book is show you the principles of skillful means in the practice of weight control. I plan to do this by showing you how to focus your awareness in a certain way. When your awareness is properly focused, weight control will be a cinch. I will show you how to see the problem in a new light and how to design strategies that will enable you to control your weight while never being hungry and always having good tastes.

I think it will help if you view this book as being about learning the skill involved in playing a game. For it is a skill we are learning, and playing is what we are doing. I think life should be fun and should be as much of a game as possible. Minimize struggle, maximize pleasure! Weight control should be viewed as a noncompetitive game in which you can, if you like, let your imagination run loose. Played by the rules, it will certainly be a very positive, energetic experience that will make you feel as if you were playing your favorite game or enjoying whatever your favorite pastime may be. It is essential to remember that with practice, the skill used in playing a game will strengthen. It gets easier. You start to do the thing naturally. At first you make mistakes, but as you keep at it, any difficulties that are first experienced will disappear as the skill becomes more and more automatic and the game becomes more enjoyable and more satisfying.

I am going to explain both the basic principles of painless weight loss and weight maintenance and the tactics I have used to successfully implement these principles. The principles are etched in stone and inviolate. My tactics can be varied, simplified, supplemented, disregarded, or otherwise refined to suit your personal tastes. The tactics are personal. While I will outline a complete set of instructions as to what you can do practically, once you understand the underlying principles, you can disregard or vary these instructions as you prefer. In effect, by following basic principles, you are going to create your own plan to suit yourself, which may incorporate all or part of my tactics, all or part of different diets or different ideas. You will only be successful over the long run when you are acting in accord with your own nature, your own plan—not someone else's nature or someone else's plan. Let me hasten to add there is no effort, no extra work required. It will all unfold as you go about your daily life. Once you see the path, following it will come naturally.

I am going to tell you things I know to be true. They work. I have used them successfully. You and I are essentially the same. Our similarities are much greater than our differences. I have experienced every kind of barrier to weight control that people experience except those that are due to glandular, metabolic, or other body uniquenesses. I know the emotional problems blocking effective weight maintenance first hand. I have stuffed myself to the gills to suppress bouts of anger, depression, boredom, etc. I know all about eating reflexively. I did it for years. I still do. I am intimately familiar with the "I'm okay until the evening, then I just pig out" syndrome. I have an enormous craving for sweets. I have been battered by these problems and more for years, and finally I have figured out how to move around them. I still get angry, depressed and bored. I still eat reflexively. I still eat at night; I still love sweets. I never let myself be hungry, and I enjoy a lot of good, satisfying tastes.

The things I will tell you work. But you must leave yourself open to hear what I am saying. Don't prejudge! You may feel that you know a lot of what I am saying, and some of it may seem obvious, even simplistic to you. That's fine! None of this is difficult. That's why it's easy to do. But it's not enough to know something. You must know it at the right moment in the right way. Your knowledge must be organized in such a way that it will work for you. If you already know what I tell you, and you are not controlling your weight, your knowledge is not organized properly. That's what this book will do for you. It will help you know what you already know in a new way, a way that will allow you to control your weight. But you must listen and do what I suggest you do. Even if an idea sounds ridiculous at first, do it. These ideas work. You can change them later if you want to. Before you can improve upon a skill, you must learn the skill. Before Picasso created abstract art, he was a master in the skills of realism. I have at times been a past master at resistance and I know how resisting can block one from experiencing, enjoying, or learning something. So unless you have a better idea of how to control your weight that works for you, let yourself be and play my way for a while, and play wholeheartedly.

Let me tell you one thing that weight control does not require: willpower! I don't have any willpower. What weight control does require is setting your mind in the right direction. I will explain this in detail in Chapter 13, "Intention Makes It Happen." There is an enormous difference between willpower and intention. Willpower means struggle. Willpower is like the image in the children's story of the little choo-choo chugging up the hill saying, "I think I can, I think I can." Willpower may work for some of the people some of the time. It doesn't for most of the people most of the time. Certainly not for me. Setting the mind allows the thing to happen naturally. The mind takes over and does the job for you. That's how easy it is. There's no teeth gritting. It seems to have a magical quality to it. Have you ever had a problem that at first you couldn't figure out how to solve? You may have consciously dismissed it. But subconsciously the problem really grated on you. You wanted a solution. After a period of time, maybe after a night's sleep, or a day or two, possible solutions began to enter your mind. You had set your mind in the direction of finding a solution. Besides wanting a solution you did nothing. Besides reading this book and doing a few simple things I outline, you don't have to do anything special. Once you absorb the principles, you will naturally, effortlessly do what is necessary.

Before I went on diets in the past, I knew I wanted to lose weight. It grated on me. It nagged me. It made me feel uncomfortable. I would be distressed by the thought of losing control, becoming truly obese. Yet for a long time I would do nothing. I really could do nothing. I made false starts and kept gaining. Now I know that all this time I was working on my mind. Trying to get it started. But the obstacles, the imagined unpleasantness would keep obstructing me. Finally when my mind was ready, I took off like a shot. What makes it easier for you than it was for me is I can tell you how painlessly the whole thing can be accomplished, if done right. It was the fear of discomfort that stopped me, and stops all would-be weight losers. Once you can understand that there need be no discomfort, that you need never be hungry, can always have good tastes, and that this will be a positive experience, then your mind will get you started a lot faster.

I have explained the ideas outlined in this book to a number of people. They have invariably come back later and said to me, "Jon, you know, you are right." No less a severe critic than my ballet dancing teenage daughter, who when she is five pounds underweight thinks she is obese, and who automatically suspects that anything I say must be wrong; turned to me and said, "Dad, you know, you're right about that Law of Deflection stuff." (Some of my ideas I have rather grandly entitled laws, i.e., the Law of Deflection, the Law of Distraction, A Very Basic Law of Nature.) But I think you will soon agree that these ideas have such universal application that they are indeed laws of human nature.

Another idea that occurred to me was that in handling the

problem of weight control, I had developed a skill in which I was truly taking charge of my body. I had never before thought in terms of taking charge of my body. But when you think about it, isn't it frequently the sensations of the body that guide the way one acts and feels, his or her moods? Wouldn't it be something if you could take charge of your body so that, for example, you could consciously make yourself feel better when you were feeling low? To some extent I have learned to do that. Through learning to cope with the urges of my body around food, I learned a skill that empowers me to exercise more and more control over myself and thereby to deal more successfully with challenges and problems in other areas of my life. Losing weight and maintaining the weight loss without struggle will lead to your dealing more effectively with your life. The rewards are great. The effort is nothing more than reading these pages and doing a few simple, painless things.

In this book, I frequently talk in terms of we, simply because we are engaged in this undertaking together. You, me and everyone else reading this book. I am actually living through this experience with you. True, I have lost all the weight I need to and have maintained the lower limit. But I am not preaching from the mountaintop. I'm right down there in the valley with you as I keep my weight under control. We're all holding hands. I've been through it and I've gotten over the hardest part, but I'm still not home free. It helps to play a game with someone who knows it better, who can teach you the ropes. While I'm a little bit out in front along the path that we're all traveling together, soon you will be leading yourself—and others—if you so choose.

Because I'm quite sensitive to the pitfalls and pains I have experienced, I am usually very gentle. But I also know there are times when I could benefit from a whack on the side of the head to shake out some cobwebs—a shock, so to speak. So occasionally I may seem a little less gentle. Sometimes I may even engage in a little tough talk just to get the juices running. Please remember I have only one overall goal for you and for me: to feel good and to keep feeling good. You will almost immediately begin feeling good as soon as you have painlessly started to lose whatever number of pounds you determine necessary. You will maintain the good feeling by painlessly keeping your weight at a desired level. The short-term objective is to lose weight. The long-term aim is to keep it off and finally get off the depressing treadmill of gaining weight-dieting-gaining weight-dieting.

I might be cynical if someone told me that he or she was going to show me how to make something hateful, like controlling my weight, into a positive, energizing experience that could be accomplished with little effort and absolutely no pain. So many promises are made and broken. At the very least, I might think he or she was a certifiable nut, dropping acid or doing mushrooms. But if it hasn't been working well for you, or if controlling your weight is a continuing and great struggle, what have you got to lose? Do it my way until you are ready and able to successfully do it a different way. Your way! For that is what I am going to show you. How to do it, your way!

Most of the problems we face in life are caused simply because we don't know a better way of doing something, a way which exists and is easily available to us, often right under our nose. We do the same old thing the same old way. Realizing the focus of the whole problem of weight control is "Now that I'm hungry, what am I going to do?" seems obvious to me now, but it took me years to zero in on it. They don't teach the right things in school. If someone had taught me to deal with my weight as I now know how to deal with it, my life would have been enhanced considerably more than it was by many of the subjects I did study.

Thomas Edison is reputed to have once said, while trying to invent the light bulb, "I know hundreds of ways that the dang light bulb won't work." Well, I came to know lots of ways to handle my weight that didn't work before I finally learned the one that would work naturally, without any struggle.

Now let's get down to business and take our first concrete step toward a lifetime of permanent weight control. We must do concrete things to turn theory into reality. What I want you to do is to simply decide how many pounds you want to lose, and what weight you would like to maintain. Set a goal at which you believe you would feel light, move well, and look good to yourself. The table on page 18, compiled by the Metropolitan Life Insurance Company, gives suggested approximate weights for different body frames. This table is presented to give you a reference point for selecting your desired weight, if you should need one. It is simply a guide for you to use. The key will be how you feel, move, and look. Possibly the weight you select will be a little too low or still a bit too heavy. You can do the fine tuning later.

Right now, just think about how many pounds you would like to lose and how much you would like to weigh. Dwell on it for a little while. In order to keep this idea in mind, say these words slowly, twice to yourself: "I would really feel and look good if I lost _____ pounds and kept my weight at _____ pounds." You fill in the blanks.

If you are tempted to skip this little exercise because you think it is corny or unnecessary, don't. Don't resist! Say it and say it slowly. Linger on it. Not only now, but every morning when you awaken and every night before you go to sleep. As a reminder to do this, attach a note to your bedroom clock so that it will hang over the clock's face. You will probably want to know the time upon waking and as you go to bed. Having to raise the note to see the clock's face will remind you to slowly verbalize your weight control goal.

By doing this little exercise, believe it or not, you have taken two major steps toward effective weight control. You are establishing a concrete goal to head toward, and you are giving your mind a signal that you are interested in it thinking about weight control. You have begun to set your mind to thin. Honestly! You are doing something important. Since there are no lights blinking or trumpets blaring and you don't feel a bit different, I know you may find it hard to believe you've done something extremely significant. But you have! However, you must do it. Just do it, do it, do it, and keep reading.

1983 METROPOLITAN
HEIGHT AND WEIGHT TABLES

MEN			
HEIGHT **FEET INCHES**	**SMALL FRAME**	**MEDIUM FRAME**	**LARGE FRAME**
5 2	128-134	131-141	138-150
5 3	130-136	133-143	140-153
5 4	132-138	135-145	142-156
5 5	134-140	137-148	144-160
5 6	136-142	139-151	146-164
5 7	138-145	142-154	149-168
5 8	140-148	145-157	152-172
5 9	142-151	148-160	155-176
5 10	144-154	151-163	158-180
5 11	146-157	154-166	161-184
6 0	149-160	157-170	164-188
6 1	152-164	160-174	168-192
6 2	155-168	164-178	172-197
6 3	158-172	167-182	176-202
6 4	162-176	171-187	181-207

WOMEN			
HEIGHT **FEET INCHES**	**SMALL FRAME**	**MEDIUM FRAME**	**LARGE FRAME**
4 10	102-111	109-121	118-131
4 11	103-113	111-123	120-134
5 0	104-115	113-126	122-137
5 1	106-118	115-129	125-140
5 2	108-121	118-132	128-143
5 3	111-124	121-135	131-147
5 4	114-127	124-138	134-151
5 5	117-130	127-141	137-155
5 6	120-133	130-144	140-159
5 7	123-136	133-147	143-163
5 8	126-139	136-150	146-167
5 9	129-142	139-153	149-170
5 10	132-145	142-156	152-173
5 11	135-148	145-159	155-176
6 0	138-151	148-162	158-179

[4]

A Bit of Terminology

I NEED TO EXPLAIN two terms that I have created that repeatedly appear in this book: "Phantom Hunger" and the "Low Calorie Solution."

PHANTOM HUNGER. Food is a fuel for the body. Phantom Hunger describes a desire for food that arises from psychological or emotional distresses rather than from the need of the body for refueling. In my view there are degrees of hunger that run from brimful, or stuffed, to empty, or famished. Phantom Hunger is the urge to eat when one is not down near the empty level. While one is uncomfortable and thinks about eating as a way to ease the discomfort, the discomfort is not caused by an empty stomach.

I call the feeling we have when our stomach is near empty, Real Hunger. It feels a certain way. Real Hunger has specific physical signals, such as a growling stomach and a certain feeling of tension. To become aware of when you are really hungry and when you are eating due to Phantom Hunger, pay close attention to how your stomach feels, both when you begin to think about eating and when you start to eat. Is it really near empty? A good way to observe Real Hunger is to not eat for a couple of hours after a long night's sleep—especially if you are not stuffed from the day before. If all else fails, don't eat for a day, and you will begin to know what Real Hunger as opposed to Phantom Hunger feels like. With proper direction such as is offered in Chapters 9 and 15, anyone can easily learn to distinguish between Real Hunger and that Phantom Hunger aroused by psychological or emotional upsets.

LOW CALORIE SOLUTION. When I am conscious of my weight, I believe that every time I am hungry it presents a problem to be solved. The challenge of weight control is to find a relatively nonfattening solution to each problem presented by being hungry. Of course, the most nonfattening solution is to eat nothing. However, that solution does not work for most people. In fact, a key to successful weight control is to Always Eat When You Are Hungry. Thus the most practical nonfattening solution is to eat or drink something with relatively few calories. In Chapter 27, "The Mathematics of Weight control," I will discuss calories more fully. For now, it is sufficient to understand that calories are a measurement of the energy-producing value of food. The energy that is in the food we eat is either used by the body for its current activity, or if not so used, the energy is converted to and stored by the body as fat. When the amount of energy (i.e., number of calories) in a person's food is greater than the amount of energy the body currently is using, the extra energy is stored as fat, and the person gains weight. If the body uses more units of energy (calories) currently than is in the food eaten, the body draws on some of its stored fat to provide the needed energy to make up for the shortfall, and the person loses weight.

As above, when talking about degrees of hunger, when I talk about the Low Calorie Solution, it is in relative terms. A Low Calorie Solution may be a food that has 10 calories instead of 50, or in the case of a dessert, 75 instead of 500. People often say to me that something I eat (which may, for example, have 100 calories) is fattening. Well, the fact is that eating something that has 100 calories may save me from eating something else with 500 calories. Thus, the Low Calorie Solution is a term of art. It is my way of describing a method of handling a moment of hunger in a satisfying manner that is much less fattening than otherwise would have been the case.

[5]

The Problem

NOW LET US RETURN to the vital question that I left hanging unanswered on the first page of Chapter 1. Why is it that so many intelligent, reasonable people, who know they would look better, feel better, be healthier, and live longer if only they would lose weight and keep it off—don't lose this weight and keep it off? The reason is that they are *forgetful*. They forget certain vital things at that crucial moment we are focusing on: "Now that I am hungry, what am I going to do?" Yes, forgetfulness is the real reason that people don't control their weight. Forgetting is also the basis of a lot of other problems. But right now we are only interested in one—overweight. After dealing successfully with your weight, you will be better prepared to deal with other problems that are also caused by forgetfulness.

I expect that after hearing this rather extraordinary assertion that forgetting, not gluttony, lack of willpower, emotional distress, etc., is the cause of overweight, some readers think I'm nuts. All readers are probably wondering what I am talking about—and essentially asking the question, "Forgetting what?" Well, there are three things that people who want to control their weight, but can't, forget at the crucial moment of "Now that I am hungry, what am I going to do?" First, they forget the *reason* why they want to lose weight and keep it off. Secondly, they forget how *uncomfortable* they will feel physically or emotionally, now or later, if they overeat, and how much longer this discomfort will last than will the momentary pleasure they may get from eating imprudently. Thirdly, they forget how to *handle their hunger in a satisfying, nonfattening manner;* in a pleasing way that will make the urge to eat disappear just as completely as if they had handled it in a fattening manner.

To truly understand what I have just said, we need to take a close look at our bodies. We need to get in touch with our bodies. We need to see hunger for what it really is, i.e., a bodily urge. Hunger is simply a feeling in our body—an agitation, a distress, a sense of unease that our body feels. What we need to realize is that this bodily feeling can be very *pleasantly gotten rid of in many different ways.* There are a variety of ways to pleasingly satisfy any hunger urge you are feeling in a manner that will make the urge disappear as completely as if you had chosen any of the other ways. It doesn't matter which way you choose. They all work!

It is really important to hear what I am saying, to focus on what I am saying. I didn't say all the choices would taste the same. I didn't say you might not like some tastes better than others. What I said was that all the choices will pleasingly make the hunger urge go away. They will all do that equally.

And here is the bottom line. There is always a nonfattening choice that will *taste good to you,* which will make any hunger you are feeling go away. Possibly at first this choice will not taste quite as good to you as something else might. But it will taste good, nonetheless.

Truly understand what I am saying. Come to understand what I am saying by clearly observing your own body. See it for yourself. Break things down as I have broken them down. See every bout of hunger as a bodily urge that can be subdued in a lot of different ways. See that some of these ways are nonfattening. See that at least some of these nonfattening choices, either in their natural state or when prepared in a certain way, will taste good to you. When you truly understand things in the way I am now explaining them, you are focusing on the problem of weight control with a laser-like clarity. Once you see a problem clearly, you are well on the way to solving it. Seen in the way that we have broken it down, the solution to the problem of weight control simply becomes to *learn* (but really learn) which low calorie foods you enjoy and *remember* to eat one of these nonfattening choices, not something else, when you are hungry. Remembering the reason why you want to lose weight, and how badly you will feel if you don't select a nonfattening way will help remind you to choose a Low Calorie Solution to any attack of hunger, as long as you are aware that a satisfying low calorie choice exists.

But you must remember your reason for wanting to lose weight and the discomfort caused by overeating in the right way, in a *feeling* sense, not just as a fleeting mental idea such as, "This isn't good for me," or "I really shouldn't." For example, in remembering the discomfort you might remember how your stomach will *hurt* after you eat, or how *distressed* you will feel when your clothes are too tight, or whatever discomfort you experience. In remembering your reason, you might think about how it will *hurt* to have a heart attack, or how *good* it will feel to be proud of your figure, or whatever your reason may be. Remember the feeling not just the idea.

In addition to seeing hunger as a bodily urge, it is extremely useful to see weight control from the viewpoint of how the energies of our body are mobilized by or against this hunger urge. People become energized with the desire to lose weight. They feel this energy, this desire in their bodies. Motivated by this energy, they will make great resolutions. My resolve to lose weight was usually at its highest when I was full, often uncomfortably stuffed, when my clothes were feeling tight, or even worse, when the buttons didn't close. "I'm going on a diet," I would grandly growl. Or more often, I would piteously moan, "I've got to go on a diet." Then what happened was that either before the diet started, or after a brief try, or even after successfully reaching a predetermined goal, I would forget the desire that moved me toward weight control.

The energy motivating my resolution had been

dampened. Other stimuli acting on me had diverted my energy from weight control. The diversion of my energy had caused me to forget what I wanted to do. I had forgotten my desire. I had forgotten the way that I felt when I made my resolution. Even though I knew in a vague way I should be acting to control my weight, now I didn't feel like doing it. I didn't have the energy to deal with weight control. It takes energy to do things. My energy was now being directed by an impulse that was devilishly pushing me to eat.

What is generally called resolution, willpower, enthusiasm, or motivation is really a form of bodily energy that a person feels pointing him or her in one direction. The impulse to chuck it all and pig out is also energy, but turned in a different direction. Most of what we actually do in life, as opposed to what we think we would like to do, is due to our mechanical responses to urges of our body. When the body is directing our energy via its impulses, if not forewarned and forearmed, we will immediately dance to its tune no matter how resolved we may feel to implement a grand plan when the body is not calling. Implementing any plan we have for ourselves that conflicts with an established pattern of behavior requires that at a crucial moment, we remember that plan and we have the energy to act. We must have another choice available—something other than what we do habitually, and we must have the energy to act in a new way.

A part of our weight control plan is to deflect any bodily impulse that is directing us toward eating more calories than we intend to, until we can redirect our energy toward the goal of controlling our weight. Now of all the ways that are proposed to deflect the urge to eat, such as walking, running, taking a cold shower, visualization, or getting involved in something to get your mind off your stomach, there is no better way of deflecting or distracting this urge to eat than to eat or drink something. Once the urge to eat has been subdued, it is relatively easy to direct one's energy back toward controlling one's weight. This is why the first commandment of effective weight control is to Always Eat When You Are Hungry. What is obviously crucial is that you remember to eat foods that are low enough in calories so that your calorie intake is less than your body's calorie expenditure. (In Chapter 7 "The Solution - Part II," I will show you how to do this.) By always remembering at the crucial moment of "Now that I am hungry, what am I going to do?" those three things that I am suggesting (why you want to control your weight; that you will feel worse if you eat imprudently than if you don't; that there is a Low Calorie Solution), and always eating to quell your hunger, you are implementing a plan that will continuously direct your body's energies as you want them to be directed—toward weight control. Not as the body had previously learned to direct them. (While this book is not about controlling the energies of the body, weight control is a form of controlling the body's energies. When this is truly understood, dealing with weight control becomes a springboard for dealing with other problems that arise from habitually yielding to bodily impulses.)

What I am telling you is to watch your body. Get in touch with your body. Take a step back and see the bodily urge of hunger as I have broken it down—as something that can be pleasingly satisfied in a number of different ways. See your motivation as bodily energy that will ebb and die if not shielded against other forces by always eating when you are hungry, and if not constantly revitalized by remembering the reason why you want to lose weight and how badly you will feel if you eat imprudently.

Now all this may sound as plain as the nose on your face, and it is. But people frequently miss the forest for the trees. I know that I did for years. The answer to difficult problems is often lying about right under one's nose. It is simply the ability to see the solution that is missing. I'm telling you something that you may think you already know, but I am telling it to you in a way that it has never been told to you before. Hear it as I am telling it, not the way that you think you may know it. The way in which one knows something affects their ability to use the knowledge. McDonald's grew from one hamburger stand to a colossal corporation with thousands of outlets in a few years by selling hamburgers and french fries. People have been selling hamburgers and french fries for decades, but the people at McDonald's had a different way of doing the same thing. They organized things in a different way. I am telling you how to organize your thoughts in a different way; how to approach your weight from a different point of view. From a point of view that truly helps you go directly to the core of what you are trying to do. People do not change because they learn new things nearly as often as they do because they see things they already know in a different way.

If you have the intention to lose weight, once you truly understand that the problem is forgetting at the crucial moment, why you want to lose weight; that you will feel worse if you don't choose a Low Calorie Solution than if you do; and that a Low Calorie Solution will satisfy the urge to eat just as effectively as a fattening one, then controlling your weight will follow naturally.

How to remember at the crucial moment and how to think about what to eat are the subjects of the next two chapters.

[6]

The Solution - Part I

HUMAN MEMORY is a basic ingredient of civilized life. If we did not remember how to do something we have once learned, we would have to relearn how to do the same thing again and again. During childhood in particular, but also throughout life, humans are learning new skills and new ideas that must be remembered in order to be utilized repeatedly. If we had to constantly relearn skills like talking, reading, and writing, civilized life would be impossible. Without memory we couldn't live on the most primitive level.

Yet human memory is really very fallible. We remember only an infinitesimal amount of the things to which we are exposed. Within days, all but the basic structure of a movie or book that has absorbed us will fade from memory; and within months or years, if we are not somehow re-exposed to the movie or book by seeing, or reading it again, or by talking about it periodically, even this basic structure will often fade into oblivion. Conversely, anything we are constantly exposed to will usually keep popping back into our mind.

Essentially, skills and ideas that stick with us do so because they are reinforced until they reach a point of being ingrained into us. Then they become habits. Habits are simply kernels of memory. And even ingrained skills and ideas must be reinforced from time to time or the habit will fade and may eventually die completely. Skills are reinforced by performance, while many of our most basic ideas are continually reinforced in our memory, in large part, through the use of symbols and rituals. While we don't usually think of these symbols and rituals as reminders, and while they also have other functions, one of their major roles is to keep us in touch with some idea or feeling.

For example, the American flag, which we constantly see, is a symbolic reminder of our national allegiance, while the playing of the "Star Spangled Banner" is a frequently practiced ritual that serves the same purpose. Reciting the Pledge of Allegiance is another ritual that serves to remind of American values and our national allegiance. Celebrating holidays such as the Fourth of July, Veterans Day, and Memorial Day, are annual ritualistic reminders of our national feelings, which also remind us of the sacrifices of particular individuals who have made a special contribution toward building and maintaining our way of life. We are taught as children to honor our values of liberty and free government. Then throughout our lives, through the use of symbol and ritual we are kept in touch with these values, and the importance of defending them.

Another prevalent source of symbol and ritual are organized religions. The cross and star are familiar examples of religious symbols that remind people of their spiritual beliefs. Continuing rituals, such as daily, weekly, and special holiday services also keep people in touch with their religious feelings. The Moslem custom of stopping to pray seven different times each day and touching one's forehead to the ground is an excellent example of a constant reinforcement of man's faulty memory.

Besides national and religious symbols and rituals, there are lots of other reminders used in our society. One example is those slogans and jingles created by advertisers to remind people of some commercial product. A second example is one person contacting another on a business or social basis for what is in large part simply an "I want you to remember

me" call. The old adage, "out of sight, out of mind" speaks
to the fallibility of human memory.

What is most on one's mind gets attention. And being exposed to constant reminders is one way to keep something
on one's mind. The secret of permanent weight control is to
remember at the critical moment of "Now that I am hungry,
what am I going to do?" those three essential ideas discussed in the last chapter: (1) why you want to lose weight;
(2) how badly you will feel physically or emotionally, now
or later, if you eat imprudently, and how much longer this
bad feeling will last than will any momentary pleasure you
may experience; (3) there is a nonfattening solution to your
hunger that will satisfy your urge to eat pleasurably and just
as effectively as will a fattening one. What we are going to
do is to place these three ideas in the forefront of our minds
so that we will remember them at the right time. Once you
have done that, you are going to find that managing your
weight is not only going to be easy, it is also going to become a stimulating, fun experience.

We know that the mind works by association. Once we
focus on an idea, a series of related ideas also come to mind.
All memory systems are based on this principle. One example is the use of notes by a platform speaker as reminders of
the things he or she wants to speak about. The notes, possibly key words, possibly short phrases, trigger in the speaker's mind those examples, ideas, anecdotes, and jokes he
wants to share with his audience. Another example of association at work would be a note to ourselves to "call Jim."
Seeing the note will bring to the forefront of our mind all
those things we want to talk to Jim about.

We are going to make the urge to eat, work for us and not
against us, by using the mind's natural tendency to associate.
We are going to make the urge to eat elicit from us the three
vital remembrances: "I want to lose weight because _____"
(you fill in the blank); eating fattening foods will make me
feel a lot worse than not eating them; that I can handle my
hunger in a satisfying, nonfattening manner. In order to
arouse this memory at the right moment, we need simply to

create a few symbols and to observe a few rituals to serve as reminders. It really is that easy. If you will consciously do what I suggest in this chapter, you will soon be on the path to a lifetime of freedom from the agonies of overweight.

The first ritual you should observe faithfully is this: at the beginning of every meal, close your eyes and say slowly and quietly to yourself twice, "During this meal I will remember that I want to control my weight because _____ (you fill in the blank); that I will feel badly if I overeat and I do not want to continue eating after my stomach is full; that I want to choose the Low Calorie Solution available." Before eating any snack, slowly ask yourself twice: "Am I really hungry? Is this the Low Calorie Solution?" Remember, you must say each of these things very clearly and very slowly, twice, so they will seep in. Don't rush through them. If necessary write them down on a card and read them until you have unfailingly committed them to memory.

Don't let there be any excuse for not practicing this ritual faithfully. If you are with someone else, turn away if it is embarrassing, or if necessary, excuse yourself and go to a restroom or some other place, and recite the words. This is a simple thing to do. Say these words unless you have a better idea than mine. If you don't practice this ritual, you need to question whether you really want to lose weight. If you don't sincerely try something as simple as this, then you probably need to give yourself a whack on the side of the head to shake yourself up a bit. If you are resisting doing this simple act or any of the other suggestions in this chapter, before reading on, skip immediately to and read Chapter 13, the chapter on intention.

The purpose of this ritual is to implant in your mind as the critical moment approaches, the idea of the Low Calorie Solution. This momentary pause, this moment of consciousness, this setting yourself in a nonfattening direction as you begin a meal or snack, will in time naturally lead to your eating in a way that will result in your controlling your weight. You don't need to learn anything to do this exercise. You need only say, whenever you are about to eat, as many say grace at the beginning of each meal, a few easy sentences. They don't even have to be my sentences. You can choose your own words. But make sure you are saying the same thing I am. By saying these words you are directing your consciousness toward weight control.

Eating normally is almost totally habitual. What you must do is arouse a consciousness while you are eating that will direct you to weight control. It is the *right thought at the right moment* that will eventually start you down and keep you going along the path of permanent weight control. Never again begin to eat without repeating these sentences. Do it sincerely and it will work for you.

We shall also create a symbol. Our symbol will be a large index card with three sentences printed on it in red letters:

1. You want to control your weight because_____ (again, fill in the blank);

2. You will feel worse if you overeat than if you don't;

3. You will choose the Low Calorie Solution.

Put one of these index cards on your bathroom mirror at eye level so that it will always get in your way; so that you will have to duck or stand on your tiptoes to see yourself completely in the mirror. It will be a real irritant and you will want to tear it down. Don't! Other people in the house will complain. Let them! That's all to the good. The quicker you lose weight, the quicker you will be able to get rid of this abomination. Let everyone else in the house cooperate with you in getting the weight off.

We stand in front of the bathroom mirror for extended periods of time doing habitual, repetitive acts that require no thinking, such as brushing our teeth and combing our hair. During this time when your mind is uninvolved, the card, like the voice of a teacher or a coach instructing you or rooting you on, will direct you toward doing what you want to do. Even if your mind wanders away from the idea of weight control, as it will most often do, the card will have an incalculable reminder value. It will continually bring you back to weight control.

This card is, in effect, you telling yourself what to do.

That's how you will make weight control work. By telling yourself what to do. That is how we make anything work. We are just not always conscious of it. We tell ourselves what to do. This card is like you stepping outside of yourself and giving yourself the directions you need.

Put one of these cards on your refrigerator door and on the door of your pantry. It will serve as a reminder anytime you are reaching for food. If you drive to work, put one on the dashboard of your car. At your job, if possible, put one at your workspace. You might put it in a drawer or on the inside of the door of a locker you open frequently. Place the card in a way that you see it every time you open that door or drawer. I realize that every reader will not be able to do the same thing in regard to these cards. Find places to put these cards where you can't fail to see them.

You will frequently ignore these cards. You may get angry at them and want to tear them up. But the message will get through. It may take a while, but it will get through to you. This is the essence of mind control—to be continually exposed to one simple message. This is what totalitarian governments do to control the minds of their people. They constantly repeat a simple message. This is what advertising agencies try to do with slogans and jingles. Human beings are extremely suggestible. Humans will readily accept suggestions that don't conflict with some preexisting, deeply held conviction. And your message to yourself is not in conflict with but is rather supporting your basic desire.

Another ritual you should practice faithfully is to carry this book with you as much as possible. Just seeing it will bring your mind back to weight control. Reread a couple of pages each day. Reread it, if you like, from beginning to end, or fold down pages you especially like so you can readily find them. Reading this book and then putting it in a drawer or on a shelf is not utilizing it most effectively. Eventually, you will forget it. Get your money's worth. Reading this book for a few minutes each day, as people read the Scriptures to keep in touch with their spiritual beliefs, will serve as a powerful reminder, keeping you in touch with your desire to control your weight. The best reader is a rereader. The ideas in this book will keep popping into your mind at the right time if you continuously expose yourself to them.

There is another very important reason for keeping this book near you and rereading it. We all need validation for our efforts, and unfortunately, we don't always get it from those around us. Know that I am your friend, your diet soulmate. Understand that I really understand. I am going through this with you and so are many others. Life can be a lonely experience. But we are all in the same boat. Let me be your constant helper, and know that I salute your actions and your successes. Also know that your successes validate me in writing this book. While we may never meet, we are helping each other.

At first, you must tend these rituals as you would a little child or young plant. They require attention and care. When they grow, they take less care. Finally, they take care of themselves. Eventually the message of the rituals and symbols will become more and more ingrained within you. But the rituals and symbols may not take hold immediately. Stay with it! Don't quit! They will do the job. Just let them! There is nothing else you need do. You simply need to keep *directing your attention to weight control* and then adopt a non-interfering attitude. If you will just keep these ideas in consciousness, your mind by itself will eventually create the energy you need to succeed. If the desire is there, the reminders will arouse you. They will take hold and when you begin to have successes, the reminders, along with the successes, and the understanding you are getting from this book will combine to guarantee your reaching and maintaining your weight goal.

Remember, in this book, I am outlining both basic principles and my personal tactics. The basic principles that will guide you to successful weight control are simple, but inflexible. The tactics used to implement the message are totally flexible. The basic principle of this chapter is to bring the idea of weight control to your consciousness as often as possible and especially at the critical moment when you are going to eat. We want to constantly direct our attention to weight control. It is important to hear the ideas over and over again, to think about them again and again, and to try and act from them.

Our enthusiasm for a thing wears off if it is not somehow reinforced, regenerated, or reinvigorated. Enthusiasm that is not reinvigorated will be overwhelmed by the diversion of our energy to other pursuits by new stimuli, which are constantly bombarding us. There are innumerable contestants vying for our energy. The way to hold onto the enthusiasm for weight control is to continuously bring to mind the ideas that encourage it. Having the right idea on center stage at the right moment is what will make weight control work naturally.

The exact words of the message can be your own. If you have a message that works better for you than mine does, don't hesitate to use it. How you bombard yourself with your message will vary depending on your individual lifestyle. The point is to have a message and expose yourself to it constantly, particularly as you begin to eat. But until you can confidently devise your own tactics, faithfully adhere to those I have outlined.

To begin implementing the principle outlined in this chapter, you must get in touch with the reason why you want to lose weight. During the next five minutes, think about it. Then write down your reason or reasons on a piece of paper. Don't put off doing this exercise until later. Do it now!

Be in as close touch with your reason as possible. Dwell on it. Use feeling words in your reason like, "I will hurt if I get diabetes or heart disease," not simply, "I don't want to get sick." Even see if you can create the feeling of your reason. Try to imagine how it would feel, for example, how good your body might feel to be thinner. Or how pleased you would feel to look better. How much you don't want to get sick, or how lousy it will feel to be sick. If you can't create the feeling, that's okay. Just know your reason and write it down.

Again, don't skip over this exercise. Do it! Simple acts that direct your mind to remembering the right thing at the right moment are what is going to make weight control happen effortlessly, naturally: simple acts, not big dramatic events. Get away from the drama of this being an ordeal, a big deal. Simply being in touch with the right idea at the right moment, and being in touch with your body will lead to your melting the pounds away for good.

[7]

The Solution - Part II

A NECESSARY INGREDIENT of enjoyable weight control is to remember to use a Low Calorie Solution when hunger strikes. The urge to eat can be satisfyingly made to disappear in numerous ways. Some of these ways will be less fattening than others. While it is absolutely essential to eat whenever hungry, what you eat must come mostly from the category of less-fattening foods.

Thus you need to know which low calorie foods are satisfying to you. Not to me, but to you. There is an appropriate adage that fits here: "One man's meat is another man's poison." Successful weight management, while following certain basic rules, is a very unique, personal experience. It is your tastes that must control. You tailor-make your own diet. Nothing else can possibly work for any extended period of time. Diets of cottage cheese and grapefruit, all protein, high fiber, or what have you, may work for a while, but you won't stay with them very long. You can't! They are not you. If you don't like the tastes, you will lose some weight, and then probably go back to old habits that will result in your gaining back the lost pounds—plus.

You begin the process of coming to know which low calorie foods will do the job for you simply by starting to notice which low calorie foods you like. Write them down. Buy a small notebook and carry it with you in a pocket or purse.

List the low calorie foods you like in this notebook. Write an idea down as soon as you get the thought or you may forget it. Don't just make a mental list. You make things happen by making them real. You make things real by making them concrete. Don't make this an abstract mind game that will fade away. Buy a real notebook and make a real list that will last. Appendix A contains nearly fifty low calorie foods that you could eat in large quantities without fear of gaining weight. Look at this list and put a check next to those foods you like (not necessarily love) either in their natural state, or when prepared in a nonfattening way. Put a second check next to those you really enjoy. The fact that you may feel you enjoy other foods more than these is irrelevant. Just think about which of these foods you feel have a pleasant taste. Begin your written list with these foods. Take some time and really think about it.

Next, start looking around for new additions to your list of satisfying, nonfattening foods. Take a close look at the calorie guide at the end of this book to get some ideas as well as to familiarize yourself with the fattening effect of different foods, particularly those you eat in large quantities. Try new foods and new combinations of foods. In the grocery store there are many calorie-reduced packaged foods. You may not like most of them, but find those you do. There are frozen diet meals, fruits, jams, dressings, snacks, drinks. And there is now calorie count information on the labels of many packaged foods that are not advertised as low or reduced in calories, and in which the calorie content is relatively modest. Read labels. Also, many of the magazines displayed near the checkout counters of most grocery stores contain articles about diets and low calorie recipes. Browse through these while waiting to pay for your groceries. A greater number of periodicals that could have helpful ideas can often be found on special magazine shelves in many grocery stores. Stop at these shelves, as you would at the vegetable or meat counter to see if anything tempts you. Spend a few minutes every time you shop, browsing through periodicals, looking for Low Calorie Solutions.

There are many cookbooks chock full of low calorie recipes. See what they have to offer. You don't have to buy one until you find a book you like. Just keep looking. I am not saying that you are going to like many of the diet ideas or recipes that you examine. I don't like almost all of them. What you are looking for are a few good ideas that will satisfy your palate. If only a very small percentage of what you think about, and are exposed to, turn into satisfying, nonfattening food ideas, then the list of foods that you can enjoyably eat when an attack of hunger strikes will be much longer than necessary.

Compiling a list of pleasurable nonfattening foods and food combinations will be an interesting, creative, insightful experience. This compiling process will also serve as another ongoing reminder that will help stimulate the appropriate memories outlined in Chapter 5 at the critical moment of "Now that I'm hungry, what am I going to do?" There isn't much to do in compiling this list. Just set your mind on the track of doing it. Give your mind the problem and it will do the work. The ideas will flow. Once you set your mind on a task, it magically takes over and starts to turn out solutions. The only thing you need to do is write these solutions down!

I can tell you that the path exists and point you toward it. But you must start walking down the path to make anything happen. There are lots of low calorie foods and food combinations that you will find truly tasty that will satisfy any hunger you may have in a nonfattening manner. But you have to go out and find them. They will not be chocolate ice cream sundaes, or chocolate cake with chocolate ice cream on top. You can't control your weight eating those things (certainly not in any large quantity). But there are lots of low calorie taste treats that can make you forget your cravings for such fat-producing goodies.

You really can get as much enjoyment from low calorie foods as from fattening ones. I once heard a slim, trim friend of mine being berated by his very overweight daughter. She told him, "You don't like food. You have no passion for food." My friend responded patiently, "That's not true. I can get every bit as much enjoyment from low calorie foods as you feel you are getting from rich foods. You just don't know that yet, because you haven't done it." My friend was right. His daughter didn't know, and she was using her erroneous, preconceived notion that low calorie foods and food combinations can't taste good, and be just as satisfying as fattening foods, as an excuse for not losing weight.

One of the major facets of the skill of weight control is to learn how to make nonfattening foods taste good to you in a nonfattening manner. I think of it as "making lettuce tasty in a nonfattening manner." It really is possible and it really is simple. You just need to think about it. I will tell you how I do it in Chapter 23.

For now, understand that it all begins with compiling your list. That is how to tell your mind to start thinking about the problem. Write your ideas down so they will be readily available when you need them. Carry your list with you so that you can refer to it while food shopping and when you are hungry. Keep adding to it. Variety is the spice of life. Let the list guide you in thinking about what to buy at the grocery store; which foods to prepare for meals; what to snack on; which restaurants to go to. Put a copy of this list on your refrigerator and food cupboard doors, so it is always around to remind you that there is a satisfying, nonfattening solution to any attack of hunger, and what that solution is.

[8]

Starting—
The Biggest Hurdle

WHEN IT CAME TO DIETING and other things, I was a big league, all-star procrastinator. You know the expression, "Don't put off until tomorrow what you can do today." I always reversed it to, "Don't do today what you possibly can put off until tomorrow." How many times have I said those famous words, "I'll start my diet next Monday." Not only did this put the horror off until Monday, it also gave me complete license to gorge myself until the big, bad day came. I don't know how much weight I gained readying myself for the great ordeal soon to begin. But it was a lot. Probably at least as much as I weigh now.

Then, on how many of those big Mondays did I wake up not feeling like beginning a diet, or even forgetting my grand resolution. Well, there was always next Monday. Then there were the times that I did start, and made it to the first night, or maybe even for a whole day or two. But soon I would falter and fall back into the same, old, hypnotic eating routine. There were a lot of false starts before I really took off on one of those fifty-pound marathons. I would rationalize that I was building myself up for the struggle. Finally, things would click, and the diet would blossom. I never understood why it worked when it worked or why it didn't work when I couldn't get going. I was like an automobile engine that keeps struggling to turn over on a cold morning; one time it just happened. Finally! Now I know that during these periods of false starts, I was unconsciously working on my mind—getting it ready. Just as I am telling you to consciously work on your mind—getting it ready, setting it in the right direction.

Starting is always the first big hurdle. Starting anything that is perceived as unpleasant is difficult. People are attracted to pleasurable activities and repulsed by painful ones. It is a normal, human tendency to put off anything unpleasant as long as one can. Maybe it will even go away and not have to be done after all. The psychiatrists call this "avoidance."

As I have already indicated, I am guided totally by the pleasure principle. I'm a guy who hates pain and deplores discomfort. The weight control method I am describing in this book is absolutely painless. There are going to be plenty of good tastes and your hunger is always going to be satisfied. That's all anyone wants from eating; good tastes, and to satisfy their hunger. Remember, the only rule is Always Eat When You Are Hungry. We are not engaged in some great ordeal. This is not going to be like doing a hundred push-ups. It is all going to happen naturally. It's all going to be a game and you are going to enjoy what happens.

It takes energy to start any new endeavor. That energy can be aroused by a positive or a negative desire. Imagine you are meandering lethargically along the street, feeling blue, without any energy. It's an effort to put one foot in front of the other. Then suppose someone comes up behind you and sticks a gun in your back and tells you that you better get around the next corner by the time he counts to ten or he's going to shoot. You are instantly going to find a lot of energy to run around that corner, and the malaise you had been experiencing is going to vanish in a twinkling. That is an example of a negative desire arousing energy. A positive desire that would instantly create some energy would arise if someone told you there was a pot of gold around the corner and the first person there would get it. Wouldn't the energy flow? The same is true of the energy you need to start your weight control program. The energy is there within you, waiting to be roused. The desire that rouses it can be negative, such as you don't want to get the diseases associated with overweight such as diabetes, heart trouble, etc.; or the desire can be positive, for example, you would like to look and feel better.

Once you start, you will certainly feel a lot better, and fast. You will see results in a day or two. You will almost immediately have more energy and feel more alive. Overeating fattening foods makes one sluggish. Within a week you will look thinner and your clothes will fit better. Realize that you are walking around with the equivalent of a 5-, 10-, 20-, 50-, or 100-pound sack of rocks on your back and you are suffering the kind of fatigue, physical discomfort and stress you would feel if you were carrying a real sack of rocks. You are going to get this load off your back. Better still, you will keep it off and you will never again feel any shame over the way your body looks, nor bulge out of your clothes.

Let me tell you two little secrets. First, the energy you need to start is right now within you, waiting to be released. How do I know that? Well, if it wasn't there, champing at the bit, you wouldn't be reading this book. It is this energy that impelled you to start reading this book. Secret two is that energy begets energy. Once you feel this energy within you and really start playing the game, the energy you need builds on itself. Honest! Once you really start, there's an excitement and interest that builds momentum. It's usually much easier to continue than to start something. Once you start, the way opens up. Then you look back and wonder why in heaven's name it was so difficult to get going.

But only you can start. Neither I nor anyone else can do it for you. I can give you a list of reasons to start, a list that you can't disagree with and can probably add to. I can show you how to do the thing. I can be with you all the time via this book, helping you handle the problems and pitfalls. But I can't do the thing for you. Only you can!

However, I can tell you from long experience that the best

time to start is now. Not tomorrow, or Monday, or after vacation, or what have you. Now, right this moment. The last diet I shall ever have to go on began in the middle of a Thursday afternoon.

I understand that you may not be in the mood, that you don't feel like it, that you feel as if you can't do it. I experienced all of that. Before my final diet, a friend of mine would frequently nag at me, "When are you going to start losing weight?" I would mutter something about "soon," and then cover my head and think to myself, "She's crazy." Now that my weight control experience has taught me something about rousing my energy and how to do it, it is a lot easier for me to start other things I don't feel like doing. If you are still stuck under the covers as I was, realize that all you need do is to rouse your energy and point it in the direction of weight control.

If you are not willing to start right now, you may need a jolt—a shock of some kind to release the needed energy. A gun in your back or a pot of gold around the corner. Maybe it will come from falling in love. Maybe you'll need to get ready for a beach party. Hopefully it won't come because of a health problem. Maybe you can think of the jolt you need and make it happen. But even if you don't think you can jolt yourself, if you will keep doing those things I am suggesting in this book, you will just start one day. The jolt will come, and once you begin to control your weight, you will feel better than if you took a vacation; it won't cost a cent, and the good feeling won't wear off.

Even if you're not ready to take the step yet, keep reading so you will be ready when the big moment comes. In the next few chapters, I will show you a fun little game and a couple of nifty tricks that will make controlling your weight a lot easier.

[9]

Awareness
Makes It Possible

A SKILLFUL WAY TO BEGIN dealing with the challenge of
weight control is to get in touch with your body; to focus
your attention on what is going on with your body in relation
to food; to notice the feeling of your body in relation to food.
Awareness is the first step to change. When we become aware
of something, we may be able to change it. Awareness makes
change possible. It requires intention to make change happen.
(I'll talk about intention in Chapter 13.)

Most of us don't spend much time observing ourselves.
It doesn't seem to come naturally, and we are not taught or
conditioned to do it. Yet, it can be a rewarding experience
that will provide insights into ourselves that can be of great
use. In order to get the ball rolling in this process of focusing awareness on how your body feels in relation to food, I
am going to pose certain questions for you to answer,
when you begin to eat, and while you are eating. The list of
questions is not necessarily complete. You may notice
other things that are of interest, and you may go into
greater detail in any of the areas explored by my questions.
Just like everything else in this book, the questions are designed to set you on the path, to get you going. Then, if
you want, you can tailor-make the processes or suggestions
to your own tastes. But by initially following my suggestions, you will understand what it is we are doing. With

this understanding, you can then, if you feel it necessary, make changes that suit your needs.

It will be extremely helpful if you write down your observations. To record these observations, use the Food Awareness Inventory on Page 49 as a guide. Make up your own similar forms and answer the questions that are asked. We tend to forget things and having these notes will preserve your impressions. Then you can review your observations and set your mind working from the foundation of your prior impression rather than starting anew. First observations are often only an overview. As we repeat an observation process, we see greater and more subtle detail, which gives added insight. Repeat this noticing process a number of times. With repetition, the ideas you develop about the feelings of your body in relation to food will expand and tend to pop more frequently into your consciousness. The increasing awareness will by itself begin to work toward the possibility of change.

1. How do you feel? For example, are you bored, happy, sad, depressed, anxious, full of energy, listless, lonely, angry, alive, feeling good, feeling bad? Answering this question helps you get in touch with your body. By thinking about how you feel before you eat, you will begin to see how you may be mistaking some feelings other than hunger for food as being signs that your body is hungry for food. A lot of our emotional life is experienced in our stomach. Sensations in the stomach caused by muscle tension and acid secretions that result from emotional states are frequently misinterpreted as hunger for food. By checking your emotional state and the feeling of the rest of your body, you can come to distinguish the sensations in your stomach that are merely falling in line with the rest of your body in reflecting your emotional state from those that are signs of a hunger for food. You will come to see that some of the feelings you are experiencing as hunger may be related to your emotions and energy level. In Chapter 15, I will show you ways to deal with emotional hunger and to direct and adjust your energy levels.

2. How hungry do you feel? Rate your hunger on a scale of one to ten, with ten being the hungriest. Recognizing just how hungry you feel can be a big help in deciding how to satisfy that feeling. For example, will a cup of coffee with a piece of fruit be sufficient, possibly even a cup of coffee alone? Or do you need something more substantial?

3. How much do you really want the food you are now eating? There are degrees of desire. Rate your desire on a scale of one to ten, with ten being the greatest desire. This is not the same question as how hungry you are. You may feel hungry, but not really want the food you are eating. You may desire the food you are eating but not really be hungry. The hungrier you really are, the more your desire will increase for any food. So if you are not really enjoying the food you are eating, double-check your hunger rating to see whether you may want to revise it downward.

4. What are the qualities of the foods you are now eating and enjoying, that make you enjoy them? Is it the sweetness, saltiness, texture, or some combination of these or other things? As explained in Chapter 11, "The Law of Deflection," recognizing what it is about fattening foods that you enjoy and desire will enable you to find ways of satisfying those same desires with low calorie foods.

5. Do you keep eating for taste after you are otherwise satisfied? An extreme example of eating for taste only, was me continuing to eat potato chips at a social event, or popcorn at a movie, way beyond any possible hunger, just for the taste satisfaction. Eating for taste occurs frequently in less obvious situations. I have a beautiful friend whom I love and adore who is an aficionado of fine foods. Frequently, when we go out to dinner, she is so full after eating about half of her main course that she has the remainder wrapped up to take home. However, this never stops her from then ordering a luscious dessert. Her rationale is that her main course stomach is full, but her dessert stomach is still empty.

With a rationale like that, you can well understand that she is both constantly lamenting she has overeaten and that she is many pounds overweight.

6. How much reflexive eating are you doing? Eating reflexively is eating continuously when your body is not in need of food, with little or no enjoyment of taste. It is an urge just to keep stuffing.

7. Notice how your stomach feels at different stages of your meal or snack. See if the first few bites satisfy your stomach which could well be the case with a snack. While eating a meal, check your stomach every few bites in order to get in touch with when you are satisfied.

8. When you have finished eating, how do you feel? Are you feeling stuffed, uncomfortable? Do you have to loosen your belt? Are you perspiring, flushed, hot, warm? Are you lethargic? Do you feel light of step, comfortable, satisfied, alive?

9. How do you feel fifteen minutes after you have finished eating? When I had overeaten, I would get progressively more uncomfortable for fifteen to thirty minutes after the meal. Do you think you would feel better now if you had eaten less or not eaten something that you did eat?

10. What are you eating that you like the taste of that is relatively low in calories? Appendix A contains a list of many low calorie foods.

11. Approximately how many calories did you eat at this meal or snack? The calorie guide at the end of this book will assist you in making this calculation.

12. Do you eat too fast? To check this, slow down and see if the taste of your food intensifies or becomes less appealing. If the taste intensifies, you are probably eating too

rapidly. If the taste becomes less appealing, your eating pace is probably not too rapid.

12A. Do you cut your food into small enough pieces? Do you chew your food well? We are told that eating too rapidly and the related bad habits of not cutting food into small enough pieces and not chewing well contribute to overeating. They are said to cause us to mindlessly shovel food into ourselves, well beyond the needs of our body. However, breaking these bad habits is really difficult, and fortunately, it is not necessary in controlling your weight. I should know. To some extent, I am afflicted with each of these poor eating patterns.

Awareness is the beginning of change. But awareness by itself does not usually produce change. It is only the first step. So please don't expect immediate, magical results as you notice things about yourself that you may have never focused on before. Don't be disappointed! Just keep noticing! Changes that you really want will happen naturally in time as a result of this continuing process of self-observation.

Breaking something larger into smaller pieces, as we have been doing with eating, makes the larger process more understandable, and may point out ways to make little adjustments that can significantly change the whole process. I used to be anxious about walking up and down steep, rough, rocky places such as the sides of hills or mountains. Then, as I was thinking about what I was doing, I noticed that if I watched where I put my feet, I would never fall. By watching where I placed my foot, by picking out the spot with my eyes that I was next going to place each foot, I was perfectly safe. I have discovered that many people have this fear of walking in steep, rough places. I have pointed out this little trick to a number of such fearful people, and their confidence picked up rapidly as they began to see how it really works.

The first time I realized how noticing a little thing may make a very big difference occurred when I was learning how to fire a rifle at Marine Corps boot camp at Parris

THE FOOD AWARENESS INVENTORY ©

1. How do you feel emotionally? (calm, tense,depressed, happy, sad, bored, anxious, full of energy, angry, lonely, energetic, listless,etc.)		
2. How hungry are you? (1-10)		
3. How much do you want the food being eaten? (1-10)		
4. What quality of the food being eaten do you like the most?		
5. How does your stomach feel? (comfortable, uncomfortable, full, empty): now? ½ through the meal? End of the meal?		
6. Are you eating for taste after you are full?		
7. Are you eating reflexively? (i.e., with little or no enjoyment of taste)		
8. How do you feel at end of meal? (light, stuffed, hot, etc.) 15 Minutes later		
9. What have you eaten that you like that is low in calories?		
10. How many calories did you eat?		

Island. There were four basic positions from which we were taught to fire the rifle: standing, sitting, kneeling, and lying flat on our stomachs. In each of the positions, we were taught a particular way to keep our left arm steady so that as the rifle rested upon it for support, it wouldn't waver and thus prevent the bullet from going straight toward where we were aiming. Getting into and staying in these positions hurt a lot. I couldn't properly get into any of them, and I didn't want to learn how. However, since there were a bunch of mean-looking, mean-talking veterans of the Korean War shouting at me to do it, I tried. God knows, I tried.

In the sitting position, you had to sit on the ground with your legs crossed in front of you and bend over from the waist far enough so that your left arm was perpendicular to the ground with your left elbow firmly planted against the ground for support. This was difficult for anyone who wasn't double-jointed. However, for me, it was physically impossible. I mean, I really couldn't do it. My back wouldn't bend that far.

Well, the head rifle instructor—a tobacco-chewing, Purple Heart veteran from rural Georgia kept screaming at me to bend down farther, bend down farther. But I couldn't. Finally, the frustration was too much for the good gentleman from Georgia, and he sat on my back as I was leaning forward, trying to push me into the desired position. I didn't budge. He kept leaning. I still didn't budge. Finally, after spewing forth some tobacco juice that went whizzing by my ear, he muttered out loud, "Jesus Christ, I never, ever saw anything like this."

Thereupon, he called all the recruits together in a circle around me, while I continued sitting in the same spot. He announced that in the prior year, ten thousand men had gone through Parris Island and the required sitting position had been good enough for each and every one of them. Then, pointing at me, in a voice overflowing with scorn, he said, "But it isn't good enough for this man." He said he was going to give me my own special sitting position in which I would place my elbow on my knee (something I could do), and use my knee as support for my arm. But he admonished all the other trainees that he didn't want to catch any of them using my sitting position, or else.

I was more than a little traumatized by this outburst, and by the very real problem of being able to fire the rifle well enough to get a passing grade or qualify when the big test would come three weeks later. If I didn't pass the rifle test, I would be set back, which meant having to stay at Parris Island beyond the normal three-month period. Being set back was a fate far worse than death. Either I learned to fire the rifle, never got off Parris Island, or would be dishonorably discharged—something I didn't want to happen. When we began firing real bullets at the targets, my scores were terrible. I was in a state of near panic.

Then I noticed something. One of the myriad directions the instructors had been hurling at us was, "Don't pull the trigger; squeeze it." The first twenty or thirty times I heard that direction I had no idea what it meant. What was the difference between pulling and squeezing the trigger? In fact, there was an enormous difference. The normal inclination is to pull the trigger of a rifle firmly. It is a natural thing to do. To squeeze the trigger meant to just apply a very little pressure, just enough to gradually but steadily move the trigger back until it reached the point of going off. In fact, the going off was actually a surprise, since you didn't know exactly when it would happen. The effect of squeezing rather than pulling the trigger was dramatic. When I squeezed the trigger, instead of pulling it firmly, the rifle didn't waver at the critical moment and the bullet would come close to the place that I aimed. My scores improved tremendously. I passed the test. All that pain of learning to get the rifle into a firm position was truly unnecessary. It could probably help to make you a somewhat better marksman, but it was possible for me to be proficient simply by noticing that squeezing rather than pulling the trigger made a vast difference.

Knowing that, I could have learned to fire a rifle pretty well in a day rather than the three weeks the Marines devoted to it.

A third time that I noticed a little something which made a big difference occurred when I realized that the reason why I and everyone else who was suffering from a weight control problem couldn't effectively deal with it was simply because we did not remember some simple things at the very crucial moment of "Now that I'm hungry, what am I going to do?" The problem was forgetting.

[10]

The Law of Distraction

HERE IS A SIMPLE, ENJOYABLE LITTLE TRICK that helps to slow down the rate at which we eat, and limits the amount of food we consume. This trick arises out of the Law of Distraction, which states that if you are deeply involved in something, time flies, the energies flow, and hunger vanishes. Certainly, Phantom Hunger vanishes when you are into something in an intense and passionate way.

The trick is to distract yourself when you are eating. If you are dining or snacking alone, one of the easiest ways to distract yourself from the food is to read something. But not just anything! You need to read something that grips you. Maybe it's an Agatha Christie or Robert Ludlum novel; maybe it's Playboy or Playgirl; maybe it's the financial or sports page; maybe it's Plato; maybe it's the Bible. You choose it. When eating alone, always come to the table with something to read, something you are really into. Of course books, magazines or newspapers are not the only possible distractions, but they are easy to carry and easy to obtain. A gripping TV program or video movie that scares you or moves you would also do the trick. But such programs and movies are just not always available when we are eating.

Essentially, in reading a compelling book, or otherwise occupying ourselves, we are focusing attention on something other than food. This focusing of attention away from food will naturally slow down our eating, and also because we find the material so gripping, rouse up our energy. The aroused energy will diminish the appetite. Notice that when you are really excited or involved, food is of little or no interest. How you are too excited, too busy, to eat. We want the mealtime to be a very positive experience, but one during which we don't overeat. Applying the Law of Distraction will help you feel alive, vital, and good, not deprived, after a meal or snack during which you have moved toward, not away from, your weight control goal.

Of course, if you are eating with someone else, reading would most probably be inappropriate. In that situation, do a lot of talking. I mean a lot of talking, as constantly as possible. And talk about something that really excites you. Maybe it's the candidates for political office. Maybe it's a movie, TV show, or book. Maybe it's your weight control program. It may be more difficult for you to talk than it would be for you to read, depending on whom you are with and whether your normal inclination is to listen rather than to talk. I am essentially a listener. My father would tell me, "Count to ten before you say something." My mother used to counsel that people would always know the kind of person you were by what you said. With that kind of early instruction, I'm usually pretty quiet unless I'm sure I have something to say that I have decided is valuable enough to utter.

However, even if you are not usually a talker, you will find that the subject of weight control will get a lot of attention. It is on a lot of people's minds. It is estimated that at any one time, 20 percent of the population of this country is on a diet. And everyone knows someone who is either coping with his or her weight or who they think should be. If nothing else readily comes to mind, talk about your weight control program and about this book. There are a lot of interesting ideas in this book that will hold people's attention. Remember that the principles of controlling weight can be directly applied to controlling other problems in life. Again, the idea is that in talking, as in reading, you distract yourself from eating; slow your eating down; and rouse energy that will dampen your desire to eat. And of course, you can't eat and talk at the same time.

One thing that I want to make clear is that distraction is only going to work up to a point. You are not going to distract yourself out of Real Hunger and you should not be trying to do that. Real Hunger is the most basic of human urges. We are not trying to distract ourselves into starvation. We are trying to distract ourselves from Phantom Hunger; that urge to eat or keep eating when we are really not hungry, when eating more would really be unnecessary, uncomfortable, and unhealthy.

But if you want to see your consumption magically and painlessly diminish, use the Law of Distraction. Read or talk while eating, or do anything else that gets your mind away from the table and gets your emotions and energies percolating.

[11]

The Law of Deflection

I AM AFFLICTED WITH a gargantuan sweet tooth. For many years, dentists have been reaping the benefits of this malady. During a nutritionally ill-spent youth, I would eat chocolate candy, chocolate cake, chocolate ice cream (frequently with chocolate syrup), and drink chocolate milk independently or often in some hideous but sinfully sweet combination. As I grew older, my sweet tooth formed a single pointedness. While once started, I could still ravage a chocolate layer cake or a large bag of M&Ms, it was toward ice cream that my yearning for sweets relentlessly drove me. I was almost always ready to eat ice cream.

One of the many moments I often literally craved ice cream was following lunch or dinner. This desire was not conceptual. It was a real, experiential, visceral, bodily desire that I felt. I didn't just think I wanted ice cream. I really wanted ice cream. There is a difference between thinking you want something in your mind and wanting it so much that your body is almost shaking with desire. The difference might be explained this way. Let's say it is just after the main course; dessert time. When one reacts conceptually, one's thought process might go something like this:"Let's see, it's time for dessert. I'll have some dessert. What shall I have? Oh, ice cream sounds like a good idea." When one reacts experientially, one just says, "I want ice cream," and heads toward the freezer, ice cream store, or calls the waiter or waitress to order it. One's body has sent a clear message to one's consciousness rather than one's mind having to create the idea.

Some time ago I began to think about my craving for ice cream and I came to realize that what I was mostly seeking was not so much ice cream, in itself, but essentially the quality of sweetness that ice cream offered. While it was also true that I liked the creamy texture and the coldness in combination with the sweetness, basically, I was just seeking a shot of relief for my sweet tooth, which apparently was activated by eating the meal before. As I mentioned earlier, I used to drink black coffee without any sugar. One day after a meal, when I was wanting some ice cream badly, I decided to try an experiment: I put some low calorie sweetener into a cup of coffee and drank it. Lo and behold, do you know what happened? I no longer wanted the ice cream. That, for me, was an eye-opening discovery. I had found a way to handle one of my greatest problems. Just a little thing done at the right moment was going to painlessly, calorielessly deflect my urge to have ice cream or any sweets. Now whenever I crave sweets and I don't want to have them, whether it is ice cream at the end of a meal or some between-meal treat, I think about deflecting that urge. I put a low calorie sweetener or possibly even a spoonful of sugar into hot or iced herbal tea. (Sometimes I have a diet soda.) If I am also legitimately hungry at the moment, I may also have a piece of fruit; a peach or an apple—to help accomplish the deflection. This is an excellent way to handle the office coffee break if it is a problem. Have a hot beverage with a low calorie sweetener, and possibly also a piece of fruit.

Remember that hunger is simply a passing bodily urge that can be pacified in many different ways. One way is to eat some food you crave. Another is to eat nothing. In either of these events, the urge will be alleviated, one in a seemingly satisfying way, the other in a much longer and unpleasant way. Whichever way is chosen, the urge for the particular sensation will go away. Bodily urges are transient. They pass away. However, if you want to make weight control easy and enjoyable, the best way is a third way: Satisfy the craving in a nonfattening manner. That is what the Law of Deflection is all about.

For most people, sweets are probably the greatest single scourge preventing them from controlling their weight, but there are others. Salt, also, has an addictive draw, especially when combined with fatty, oily substances and textures such as potato chips, peanuts, pretzels, crackers, bacon, and certain hors d'oeuvres. The primary attraction of these foods is their saltiness. It is true that the texture is also a draw, but that is secondary to the attraction of the salt or, possibly, some other seasoning or taste enhancer. To prove this, notice how most people put salt or ketchup on french fried potatoes. Or try a meatball without any seasoning and taste the difference between it and one of those hors d'oeuvre delicacies that people like me keep eating and eating. Once I realized that I was mainly attracted to the saltiness of certain temptations that I could eat endlessly, I would simply take a piece of celery and put some salt on it in order to deflect and satisfy the urge that I had for the salty goodie. Now I grant you that celery with salt is not the same thing as french fried potatoes with salt. But after eating the celery with salt, I don't want french fries. Try it!

I could deflect my enormous urge for bread simply by eating raw vegetables (celery, carrots, cucumbers, lettuce, etc.) It is true that these are not much like bread in either texture or taste. But what I was really doing with bread was satisfying an urge to stuff myself, rather than responding to a compelling taste addiction. The stuffing urge might be triggered just by eating the first piece of bread or by some emotional trauma. I learned that I could kill the urge for bread simply by stuffing myself with low calorie vegetables. I would often put a little something on the veggies like cottage or ricotta cheese, just as I might put something like this on the bread.

I think the proof that my bread addiction is really a stuffing urge, and that I can deflect it by eating a lot of something else, becomes clear when I am in restaurants. In the past, I would often start eating bread the minute it was placed on the restaurant table. I would go through a basket or two before the main course arrived. One piece of bread led to another (it didn't even have to be very good bread). However, when weight conscious, as I always am now, on entering a restaurant, I immediately order a salad, eat it, and possibly order a second one. The salad or salads get me over the bread mania. Then after I eat the main course, I am full, and my interest in bread has completely disappeared.

There are many ways to prepare food in a low calorie manner that will satisfy the urges you feel to eat higher calorie foods. A personal example is the way my urge for rich, creamy foods can be satisfied by a skillfully prepared, low calorie, yogurt-based dip or sauce. Once one understands which tastes and textures one wants, it is simply a matter of thinking about, and experimenting with, ways to deflect a desire by feeding it a low calorie or no calorie substitute for the fattening food that one mistakenly believes is necessary for his or her satisfaction. Remember, when you deflect the urge, it disappears just as if you had eaten the fattening food. There is no difference. And there is no deprivation at all in deflection. When you deflect the urge, you no longer want the fattening food, and you feel good. When you don't deflect the urge and take the fattening way, you may well want even more of the fattening food. What is worse, you will probably feel badly physically and/or emotionally, either immediately or soon thereafter.

[12]

Always Eat
When You Are Hungry

THE FIRST OF THE TWO COMMANDMENTS of effective weight control is Always Eat When You Are Hungry. Knowing that you can and should always eat when you are hungry, and understanding that there are a lot of satisfying tastes available in low calorie foods, provides the security one needs to combat the idea that losing weight and weight control are an ordeal.

Once you have a firm grip on this security blanket, you are able to begin freeing yourself from the negative vibrations that the idea of weight control arouses in most of us. The idea of losing weight certainly raised a lot of resistance in me, and I believe it does in everyone. It is this negative viewpoint which makes it so hard to start and so easy to stop a weight control program. Truly knowing that you can eat food that is satisfyingly tasty whenever you are hungry makes it possible to finally have a positive point of view about weight control. Now you are in control of your hunger rather than your hunger being in control of you. You are fortified to resist the temptation to deviate.

Once you are completely confident that you can eat any time you like, you can more easily stop eating at mealtime or any other time. Leaving the table is easier if you know that you will not be without food for the next few hours and that you can put something in your mouth at any moment.

Knowing that at any moment you can eat something that tastes good will prevent the type of despair that blocks many people from starting, or leads them to soon abandon, a weight control program. There should never be any guilt about eating, because there never is a requirement not to.

The second commandment of effective weight control is that the only foods that one can eat in large quantities must be low in calories. One can most assuredly eat other foods, but these must be eaten with some discretion, depending upon how addictive the food may be, and what stage of the weight control process a person may have reached. There are plenty of good tastes available in low calorie foods alone, or in combination with small quantities of a higher calorie food that itself if consumed in too vast a quantity would seriously damage a weight control program.

At the beginning of a diet, all I ever tried to do was to get used to eating nonfattening foods. I never thought about quantities. I just kept eating until I didn't want any more. I stuffed myself. I mainly concentrated on the type of food I was eating and making it taste good. What happened was that within a day or two I began to feel better and lighter. Within a week, I realized I had lost some weight. This happened automatically while I was stuffing myself with really low calorie foods. (I concentrated mainly on vegetables and fruits. But I also ate cereals and protein.) Most importantly, within a short time, my appetite began to diminish on its own.

Within a week or two after starting a weight control program (maybe longer, depending on how excessively one eats), one will naturally start to eat considerably less. The reason is that you never needed all that food that you were putting into yourself. Once your body realizes there is no deprivation, it will start to be clear to you that you don't want as much, you don't need as much, and you are really not comfortable eating as much.

A second reason that food consumption diminishes after a while is that success breeds enthusiasm for more success. One will begin to naturally help the process along. Knowing you can eat whenever you want to, and feeling both lighter and successful, you will begin to feel less like indulging yourself. Why spoil a good thing? In time the emphasis will gradually shift from needing to feel safe by stuffing yourself to wanting to see more and more success. This tendency will increase as time goes on, but somewhat unevenly. There will still be moments when you just want to eat even though you're not really hungry. Go ahead; eat! But be sure you eat low calorie foods. There will be fewer and fewer of these moments when you are eating in response to a Phantom rather than a Real Hunger. And when you do eat in response to Real Hunger, you are going to find yourself enjoying the taste of what you are eating more than you will when eating in response to Phantom Hunger. The taste will be more intense.

Beware! You may even start to become overzealous. This is not a good idea. Don't become a fanatic. Simply find the pace that keeps you comfortably losing, and then maintaining, your weight. If you are too zealous, you create more of a challenge than is necessary. You run the danger of becoming uncomfortable. It is essential to keep the body comfortable at all times by keeping it fed.

[13]

Intention
Makes It Happen

ARENESS MAKES IT POSSIBLE to understand conceptually how a problem can be solved, but it takes intention to put the solution into effect, to actually do the thing.
It is intention that makes things happen. Intention arouses
the energy needed to do the thing! Awareness makes it possible. Intention makes it happen!

This book is teaching you a painless, proven, personal
method for getting your weight under control—but you
must have the intention to do it. You and you alone create
that intention. Neither I, nor anyone else, can create that intention for you. "You can lead a horse to water, but you can't
make it drink."

Intention is simply a state of mind. With the right state of
mind, things are easy. If you hate a task, it will be difficult to
do. If you love doing something, it will be fun and easy.
When you have intention to do something, there are no ifs,
ands, or buts. It's like telling the salesman to stop wasting his
breath. "My mind is made up." It's like a three-year old
stamping his foot, crying, "Won't, won't, won't," no matter
how much you coax him or her to do whatever he or she
has decided not to do.

Intention is not willpower. Willpower is a different state
of mind. With intention, there is no doubt, no issue. With
willpower, there is a sense of struggle. If you are trying to

develop willpower, you are leading yourself into a negative place—a place where you will feel deprivation that you will have to struggle against. Willpower will almost always fail somewhere along the way. Intention won't. Intention is beyond struggle. Intention is positive. When you have intention, you look for a solution to a problem instead of giving in. You just act in such a way that makes what you intend to happen, actually happen.

Once you really decide to do something, it is easy. Recently, I overheard a lady standing in front of me on a line at a salad bar, somewhat mournfully remark to her companion that she was starting a diet, but she didn't really know what would come of it. That woman did not yet have the intention to lose weight. She wanted to lose weight conceptually, but she didn't feel that it was going to work. Yet she was the only factor that was going to make it work or make it not work. It wasn't going to happen to her.

I know that lady's state of mind. As I related earlier in this book, I started a lot of diets that died on the vine. But once I developed the intention to lose weight, it became a cinch. Then I didn't have the slightest trouble turning from foods to which I am addicted. People remark about what they call my self-discipline, my willpower, in the face of tempting delights. Nonsense! I wouldn't even think of eating those foods. That doesn't mean I didn't at times feel a flicker of temptation. I did. But once I entered the right state of mind, not eating them was simple. I just deflected the temptation by eating a nonfattening alternative that I also enjoy. Knowing I would never be hungry and that I could find a satisfying, nonfattening taste that would alleviate the urge I felt made this intention possible.

I have described what intention feels like, and what it looks like. I am sure that at times you have experienced that kind of intention in other areas of your life. If you really want to lose weight or do anything else, the intention is there naturally, and the obstacles do fall away. The Sufis say that when you really want to do something, you develop the organ you need to do so. However, it does help to have someone urging you on, backing you up, and showing you how. That's what this book is all about.

Intention is more easily formed when the task seems quite doable, and is seen in a positive light—when the path you will follow has been successfully followed by others before you. What I am telling you is that the doing is easy. And believe me, I am nothing special. Underneath a carefully constructed exterior designed to meet the world (just as we all have an exterior constructed to meet the world), I'm a self-indulged, spoiled child. If I can do it, anybody can!

The major obstacle to my developing the intention to control my weight was my belief that I was going to suffer, that I would be depriving myself of something I really wanted. Once I came to truly understand that it wasn't painful, that there would be no deprivation, and that I was going to feel better and look better, it became easy to develop and then maintain the intention to control my weight.

While I can't develop the intention for you, I can tell you how to go about rousing it in yourself. Intention is roused by first deciding that controlling your weight really matters to you. Is controlling your weight a priority item in your life? If not, why are you reading this book? If so, the next step is to create a *magnetic center,* a nucleus within yourself that will attract you to weight control and weight control to you. You begin to create this magnetic center by paying attention to weight control. The more you think about, the more you pay attention to your weight, the easier it will be to develop the intention. You develop a commitment by paying attention, and really coming to understand in your bones that weight control is important and that it is easy. By paying attention to, and thinking about your weight, as I have been showing you, you will begin to naturally take the steps necessary to control your weight. Your body will truly wake up to the fact that controlling your weight is important. You will begin to see that you can do it.

It may take some time. Remember, we aren't talking about a diet for seven days; we are talking about a skill that will last a lifetime. I didn't just decide, one day or one minute, that I was going to control my weight. I had to feel bad, to keep thinking about it. I had to have a growling, grumbling, nagging voice inside of me asking, was I really going to allow myself to get that fat? You create enthusiasm for weight control by constantly focusing on the benefits. Think about how good it will feel. Try to imagine, try to feel how good it will feel. How good you will look. See a thinner you in your mind's eye. Realize what a relief it will be to be off that gain weight-lose weight treadmill, free of the power your food addictions now have over you.

Don't just read this book. Carry it with you. Do what is suggested. Say the things before meals, when you awaken, and again before bed outlined in Chapters 3, "Knowledge is Power" and 6, "The Solution - Part I." Buy a small notebook and make your list of nonfattening foods and snacks. Keep adding to this list. Refer back to this book. Reread parts of it for a few minutes a day. Keep a copy on your nightstand, possibly another in the bathroom, in your purse, briefcase, etc. Rereading this book will inspire you to keep your energy directed toward weight control. Scan through magazine articles and diet cookbooks for low calorie ideas. Look around in the grocery store. If you're not ready to start yet, just keep thinking about the effect the food you are buying and eating has upon your weight; and after you have eaten, ask yourself, "How could I have done this in a nonfattening way that would also have been satisfying?" Keep doing these things, and the magnetic center will keep growing, drawing you to weight control. It will all happen naturally. The intention will form. You will begin to control your weight. You will just do it.

There are those who say people who are overweight want to be overweight. I don't believe that. I think that's just a cop-out. I think most people who are overweight are that way because they don't know how to deal with the problem effectively. They don't know any other way. In essence, their intention is blocked by lack of knowledge. They are not directing themselves properly. They have drifted into certain responses to food, and they haven't found the way to change these responses without feeling pain or deprivation. They are simply stymied because they don't understand that weight control is a skill that has to be learned. They don't understand what the problem is or how simple the solution is. These people haven't felt they had permission to eat when they were hungry. They haven't learned to seek and identify those nonfattening foods they enjoy. What these people must come to know is that they really can find many nonfattening foods they like. The intention to lose weight leads one to find the nonfattening foods he or she can enjoyably eat, and to remember to eat these foods, instead of fattening foods that will only intensify discomfort. If one doesn't find low calorie foods one enjoys, it can only be because he or she isn't looking, and if one isn't looking, it can only be because he or she doesn't want to look. If so, this person must ask him or herself, why? Only he or she can answer that question. Don't make a lot of mealymouthed excuses. Stop indulging yourself. Just do the thing! Do the thing! Do it!

[14]

A Basic Law of Nature

THIS IS A VERY SHORT SECTION. It has one point to make. But it is essential to understand and to keep it in mind, especially if you are still resisting the idea that it may be possible to lose and control your weight in a painless and positive manner.

When you are really hungry, any food tastes good. This is a basic law of nature. I am sure you have noticed how particularly good food tastes when you are really hungry, how it "hits the spot." When we are really hungry, all foods taste better, even those we are not normally attracted to. For example, I hate calf's liver. But when I'm really hungry, I'll even be glad to eat calf's liver, though if possible, I still prefer it smothered in onions and doused with condiments.

My point is that if you are shying away from low calorie foods because you don't think they taste as good as some fattening delight, you are not really hungry. When you are thinking, "I'll never eat celery" (or some other low calorie food), "I hate that stuff," you're not really hungry. You will gladly eat almost anything when you are really hungry. When traveling along the path from full toward hungry, the closer we come to Real Hunger, the greater will be the number of foods that taste good, and the less power our addictions will have to make us believe the utterly false notion that only fattening foods can be tasty.

When you can't find a nonfattening taste that is satisfying, you may want food on some conceptual level, but your body is not really hungry for food. You are looking for certain tastes. This is a form of Phantom Hunger. As I have continually stressed, you should eat whenever hungry on any level (conceptual or real), but deflect the urge for those fattening tastes that are controlling you by applying the Law of Deflection, as explained in Chapter 11.

When you deflect it, the urge for the taste will quickly pass, and each time you don't succumb, the desire will be weakened. Then the urge will come less frequently, and when it comes, it will little by little feel less intense. The urge will exert less control over you. Finally, you will be free of it and feel a lot better.

Remember, when you are really hungry, there will be more than a sufficient number of nonfattening tastes that you will find very satisfying. Knowing this, truly understanding it, and remembering it will always lead you to choose a nonfattening solution to a moment of hunger.

[15]

Emotional Hunger

IT IS SADLY THE CASE that some people, including me, eat in order to seek relief from emotional distress. Frustration, anger, hurt and depression often have individually or in combination triggered me onto an eating spree. As described in Chapter 16, Reflexive Eating (a form of emotionally triggered eating), when unleashed, I would go from one ice cream store to another, buying chocolate ice cream cones, or stuff myself with bread by the loaf to try to soothe some inner distress.

Emotionally triggered eating is really a habit that some of us have. Because of our conditioning, we habitually respond to certain types of emotionally aroused energy by eating. This tension elicits an automatic desire for certain types of foods, often sweets. Maybe this comes about because, when we were children, our parents, or other authorities, would give us sweets when we were sad, in order to make us feel better. Maybe it is because when we were kids, sweets were used as treats or rewards for desirable conduct. Maybe it is because a major way our parents expressed their love was through the way they fed us. Whatever the reason, emotionally triggered eating is a big, big problem for those of us unfortunate enough to suffer this affliction.

My own childhood offers a vivid example of the way food is often used as an expression of love. My grandmother was probably the archetype of all grandmothers. She was a little, stooped lady with an incredible determination to have things work out her way. No matter what the time of day, the moment someone walked into her house, she would sit the visitor down at the big table that dominated her combination living room/dining room and upon which she would immediately begin heaping items of food. "Eat, eat, eat," she would keep saying in the Eastern European accent that she had never cast off, despite over fifty years of living in this country. If you didn't eat, she kept hammering at you, putting new things on the table, until you finally succumbed; and she didn't let up until she was satisfied you had enough.

Frequently, the women in my family would protest that they were on diets, and if they ate, they would get fat. My grandmother was always ready for such resistance. Undauntedly pressing food on the protester, with a certain irritation she would say, "In my house, there is no dieting." Then she would recount the way it was when she was a young woman in the early 1900s. In those days being chubby was considered attractive, she'd say. Men wouldn't look at women who were thin or who looked like the fashion models of today. As a kid, I thought she was making it all up, but in fact, I later found out it was true. Chubby was in style fifty years earlier.

I also later came to understand that feeding people was the way my grandmother could allow herself to express love. To some extent, that same pattern of constant feeding was the way that love and affection were expressed by most of the women in my family. When we learn to equate food with love, it's easy to overeat.

Dr. Neil Solomon, in his book, "The Truth About Weight Control," says: "People react in one of two ways to tension. They eat or they stop eating. Thin people and people of normal weight usually under tension stop eating, while fatter people tend to stuff themselves when the going gets rough." While I essentially agree with Dr. Solomon's point, I don't believe that tension alone causes one to eat. In fact, certain tension dulls my appetite. I believe that what creates my compulsion to eat in some emotionally charged situations is that at the moment I have no way of expressing the energy bubbling inside of me. The nervous energy is causing a seemingly unpleasant sensation that I am conditioned to believe food will pacify. But if I can get that energy working for me in a positive manner, handling a problem, or otherwise focused on some activity, I will be much less prone to eat. If not directed to some activity, the energy gets used in eating. When eating, I am doing something—chewing—which is a way to work off my bubbling over-energy.

When people are tense, their teeth may be clenched or may even chatter, and their jaws may feel tight. A lot of nervous energy gets worked off by the action of one's teeth and jaw. Chewing gum is a common way people have of dissipating nervous energy. Eating is another.

Also, in eating when emotionally charged, we are in effect stuffing the energy down. Notice your energy level after a big meal. How sluggish you may feel. By stuffing food into ourselves, we try to smother the emotionally aroused energy.

The best, and possibly only way, that one conditioned to respond to stress by eating can avoid doing so is to direct the swirling energy within toward an external activity. *Do something!* Choose some way other than eating to let off the steam. If possible, do something you truly enjoy. Apply the Law of Distraction. But you need to be really involved. Half-hearted, uninvolved activity like studying for an exam, probably will not work. Your interest will not be great enough to completely distract your tension from goading you into eating. Intense physical exercise is an excellent way to work off nervous energy: running, walking, or playing any sport you like.

Another emotional state that causes many people to eat is depression. I know something about depression. I have experienced my share. I think depression is caused by one's energy being turned inward toward oneself, rather than being directed outward toward the world. While one feels anything but energetic when one is depressed, there is an enormous amount of energy at work. Unfortunately, it is being directed inward and is causing intense distress. As is the case with bubbling nervous energy, some relief will be felt if the inwardly directed energy causing the depression is temporarily stuffed down with food.

The best way to handle depression is to turn the energy outward. This is easier said than done, because the last thing one wants to do when one is really depressed is to move. One wants to just lie around and mope about. One is really dragging. But we must do something that will get the energy inside moving outward. It is like the person who is stranded in the frozen Arctic who must keep moving to live. He may feel like all he wants to do is lie down and sleep, but he must move.

To overcome depression, one must simply move. If you like some sport, do it. If not, run, or just go for a brisk walk. Get that energy flowing outward. Do something! Think about what you like, and do it. If you can't think of what you like, keep thinking. Believe me, you really like a lot of things, though you may not always be in touch with what those things are.

I learned that I liked a lot of things I never thought about when a lovely woman whom I had just met asked me what I would like to do for my upcoming birthday. I replied in a then typical, phlegmatic way, "I really don't care." She responded insistingly "There are really things you would like to do. Just think about it." So I let myself think about it, and within five minutes I had a list of four things (all very reasonable and possible) that I would like to do. And as I thought about it, I became more and more excited by the idea of actually doing them.

If depression is causing you to eat, get in touch with what you like, what interests you. Don't just read these words. Think about it. Make a list of what you like. If nothing comes to mind, how about classes to learn about new things? Or how about helping others—volunteering to assist some community organization? There is always someone you can help in some way. And helping other people makes us feel good about ourselves.

I know that if you are in a depression, you don't feel like moving. But moving is all you have to do. *Move!* Get the energy flowing! Begin by simply putting one foot in front of the other. Once you get going, you find it to be easier and easier. Know that what stands between you and feeling better is simply getting your energy flowing. Flowing energy does for depression what an aspirin does for a headache. The sure-fire and possibly only natural medicine for depression is activity. And everyone can find things they enjoy doing that will make them feel good.

Another common emotional state in which misdirected energy causes us to eat is boredom. When we are bored, we usually have a lot of restless energy and nothing appealing to do with it. So one's hand goes to the cookie jar or what-have-you, in order to try to fill in the time with an artificially created pleasant experience. The positive alternative to eating when you are bored is, again, to direct the energy toward something you enjoy doing. Understand that you are bored; then simply do something.

But there still may be times, as there still are occasionally for me, when you can't focus your excess energy on some absorbing activity, or turn depression-causing energy from an inward to an outward course. The pain or frustration may be so great you can't do anything else. Then go ahead; eat. Stuff yourself if you must, but stuff yourself with nonfattening foods. Use the Law of Deflection. If you need sweets, as I do, eat foods that are sweet but have relatively few calories—fresh fruits, diet soda, coffee or tea with low calorie sweeteners. If you need to stuff yourself, do it with low calorie vegetables. Try to distract yourself first. If you can't do that, deflect your urge to eat. It will work!

The trick to handling emotional hunger is to learn to recognize the signals that the hunger you are feeling is emotional in nature and to remember what to think about in order to dissipate it in a nonfattening manner. Using the Food Awareness Inventory introduced in Chapter 9 will help you learn to recognize your emotional hunger signals, and what I am suggesting in this chapter should set you on the path to developing a strategy to dissipate emotional hunger whenever it arises.

Eventually, as you come to have some experience in recognizing and directing the energy caused by emotional upset, you will find yourself having to give in to food less and less. The first time that in a moment of stress I successfully diverted myself from eating sweets by directing my energy elsewhere was a major triumph for my weight control program. It probably signaled the fact that this time it really would be different. There would be no more gain-weight periods. The cycle was broken!

Eating excessively does not make one really happy. Eating excessively does not make one feel good. Too much food does not give lasting pleasure. At best, food offers a momentary sensation of pleasure. When eating is overdone, as with anything else, it becomes less and less pleasant, and eventually uncomfortable. Stuffing food in can ease the pain for a brief while, but it doesn't cure the problem, and it leads quickly to other types of problems. Being overfed and overweight makes people feel bad. Losing weight and feeling light makes people feel good.

When I started to remember the momentary nature of the pleasure that food gave; the much longer period of physical discomfort that followed my overeating; the feeling of being too full, heavy, lethargic; and the emotional discomfort I felt because I didn't like being fat, I was able to get my weight under control. I still have a lot of emotional stress. I still have a lot of poor habits. But now I work around them.

Another powerful thing that I came to realize was how losing weight would help alleviate emotional distress. You don't have to solve the emotional hurt before losing weight. In fact, if you are waiting to solve the emotional upset first, you can wait a very long time—possibly forever. Losing weight will help soothe emotional distress. Losing weight makes you feel good. You don't have to improve your self-image or think thin before losing weight, though such mindsets help. Losing weight will automatically help your self-image and help you think thin.

This is a very important idea to focus on. Your weight is something you can control by yourself. You don't need to rely on anyone else for help. Weight control offers a chance to be successful, to feel good about yourself, and to be in control of your life. All you need is to learn the skill of weight control. Then do the thing.

I am not saying that controlling your weight will make all the problems of your life go away. I am saying that by helping you to feel better about yourself, controlling your weight will help you cope with emotional upsets more effectively, and will tend to minimize both the number of and the intensity of these upsets. Losing weight and keeping it off will instill within you a state of mind that will spark good things happening. All this will have a very positive effect on your life. It happens magically.

I am also not saying, that depending on the circumstances, you might not additionally benefit from other forms of assistance that would help you cope with emotional problems, such as psychotherapy, counseling, or support groups. A sensitive listener, a skilled counselor, and/or one who has experienced the distresses we are going through can frequently help us deal with problems more effectively.

In closing this chapter, I'm going to mention a few ideas that help me handle emotional upsets. They don't eliminate the upset, but remembering them when I am able to, helps.

One is the transient nature of all experience: "This too shall pass." Both the good moments and the bad ones go fleeting by for everybody. And in particular while one is experiencing the bad ones, it can help to realize that everything changes.

A second is the idea of "looking for the blessing in disguise." Look for the positive aspects of every experience, and focus on them. There can be a silver lining in any cloud. Out of every experience comes something new, and what is at first perceived as bad often leads to something else that is perceived as good.

And finally, don't punish yourself. Almost all emotional

upset is self-inflicted. Obviously, there are moments of true grief in real life, but there are many more moments of self-created grief. This self-created grief usually comes about because one is down on one's self for not doing, saying, knowing, being, having, or accomplishing something. Many of us set ridiculous standards and impossible goals for our lives. Then we punish ourselves for not meeting these standards and reaching these goals. If you don't like something you are doing or saying, don't beat on yourself. Just recognize it and say to yourself, "There I go again. So what?" If you keep noticing something you don't like in this way, you will in time act naturally to change whatever is causing the distress, or come to comfortably accept yourself as you are. Maybe not the first or second time you notice it, maybe not the tenth. But in time, one or the other will happen.

While knowing these things won't offer magical momentary solutions, bringing them to consciousness at the right time can be a big help in coping with and more quickly getting over upsetting events. Most importantly, thinking of any of them at the crucial moment may well direct you away from a habitual response to food and toward a nonfattening solution to the emotionally triggered Phantom Hunger you feel.

[16]

Eating Reflexively

REFLEXIVE EATING is continuous unconscious eating beyond any possible bodily need for nourishment. A reflexive eater eats on and on because of a felt need to keep *stuffing* food into his or her stomach, or because he or she is so hooked on the *taste* of something that he or she just keeps eating even though the body has no need of the food. At times, reflexive eating begins with eating for taste, then continues, well after the taste buds become dulled due to overexposure, in order to satisfy some almost hypnotic urge to keep stuffing. When this happens, the eater is living on the memory of the taste, the concept of the taste and is just satisfying the urge to stuff. Any physically normal person who is overweight is to some extent eating reflexively. As is the case with any vice, some overweight people are much greater reflexive eaters than others, but all overweight people are doing some reflexive eating. Let me tell you about the patterns of one pretty fair reflexive eater. Me!

I ate ice cream and bread reflexively. I used to tell people I met that 90 percent of what they saw in front of them was ice cream and dough. I would often eat ice cream by the quart, occasionally by the half-gallon. I would start with a generous portion. When I had finished, without any thought I would go back to the freezer for a second, then a third, then a fourth, until I had finished the container. After a while, I really didn't know how it tasted. My tongue would become increasingly numb with the cold. Sometimes I would go from one ice cream parlor to another, buying chocolate ice cream cones. I would buy the first cone and eat it in my car as I was driving to the next ice cream shop. (I was too embarrassed to go back to the first store.) Then immediately thereafter there would be a third shop and a third cone. As for bread, I could polish off a loaf in a short time. First I would have one or two pieces. Then back again and again until the loaf was finished. I was stuffing it in and I was uncomfortable, but I kept on eating.

My reflexive eating pattern most often would be triggered by some emotional trauma—anger, anxiety, depression, boredom, frustration, etc. I would simply start with one portion of ice cream, or one or two pieces of bread. I never thought when I had the first portion of ice cream or piece of bread that I would keep going. It just happened.

I still eat reflexively at times, though much less often than before. But when I do it now, I eat nonfattening foods, such as celery, lettuce, cucumbers, Melba Toast, etc. However, knowing that I am prone to eat reflexively, I do catch myself at it. I have learned to deal effectively with the pattern. I found that it helps to drink a lot of liquids while eating, in order to help create that stuffed feeling I want. I have also learned to use the Law of Distraction explained in Chapter 10. Once I become aware of and stop the reflexive stuffing, it isn't very long before I don't feel like eating any more. I realize that I'm too full and that eating more won't feel good. A little bit of awareness can make a big difference.

Reflexive eating can be stopped dead in its tracks if you can just focus on whether continuing to eat will really make you feel better or worse. Will eating the next bite make you feel better or worse? Before having the next bite, check your stomach. When you are reaching for the second or third helping of sweet potatoes at Thanksgiving, check your stomach. Be in touch with your body.

When I am truly in touch with the fact that eating more is going to make me feel uncomfortable, the urge pushing me to eat will give in, though grudgingly. It is like choosing the lesser of two evils. But since I am really in touch with the fact that eating more will make me feel worse, and that the urge to stuff will pass, my body makes the best choice available and I stop eating. Zeroing in on the discomfort which must follow from reflexive eating will eventually lead to your stopping. Each time you notice the discomfort that follows your reflexive eating will lead to the moment that you begin to stop. It may take a number of episodes of noticing, of focusing on the discomfort, until it works. But you will eventually get the point and stop. Our bodies are not naturally attracted to discomfort. We only choose the path of discomfort because of a lack of awareness—a distortion that veils the *relationship of the discomfort from its source.* When you become able to see the discomfort that reflexive eating causes and the lack of pleasure it gives before you start eating rather than afterwards, then your reflexive eating pattern will begin to die.

To a certain extent almost everyone eats reflexively. Certainly anyone who is overweight is doing some reflexive eating. I am outlining my reflexive eating patterns so that you will know that I am a pretty far-gone case. Most people are probably not nearly as bad as I am. I probably have worse eating problems and eating habits than most of the people reading this book. I am telling about my habits so that you can have confidence that the things I am outlining in this book that have worked for me and others can also work for you.

It is important to know which foods, if any, you eat reflexively, and to be wary of them. If possible, stay away from them completely. When losing weight, I hardly ever ate ice cream or bread. If I did, I was careful to eat these things slowly and to drink something hot along with them. I would try to abstain completely and would preferably use the technique explained in the chapter on the Law of Deflection. But occasionally, because of the social situation, because I was hungry, and because there was nothing else available that I could eat, I would eat bread products or ice cream. But I would eat these addictive foods very slowly and I would drink a lot of hot liquids with them.

It is also important to understand that taste often begets desire. Eating something can make you hungry for it. You may not really need to have the first bite, but once you have had the first bite, you can't not have the second bite. With me it is ice cream and bread. With you it might be something like peanuts and potato chips. Staying away from the first bite is a lot easier than staying away from the second bite. And staying away from the first bite is really a lot easier than it may sound. Once your mind is set in the direction of weight control, not having the first bite is easy enough. Just use the Law of Deflection and avoid whatever it is that turns you on to excess; without feeling the least bit deprived.

[17]

Midstream

AFTER YOU HAVE BEGUN to successfully lose weight, but before you have reached your goal, a number of evil forces may conspire to throw you off the path leading to painless weight control forevermore. The initial energy that got you started, which received a powerful boost from your early successes will begin to wane. Energy needs to be periodically reinforced or it will slowly fade. You might see this by imagining what happens when a stone is thrown into a lake so calm that its surface is like a large mirror. The initial energy of the stone creates a series of widening ripples which will eventually vanish unless a second stone follows the first. Without a second stone to reinforce the energy which caused the rippling, the surface of the water will return to its calm mirror-like state.

Unless reinforced, the original resolution that launched your weight control program will also fade. Your program will fizzle as would a rocket into space that after a brilliant launch is not given a boost with a second stage of thrust. The novelty and pride felt at early success will begin to wear off. True you are feeling a lot lighter and that is a great feeling, but the spectacular early weight losses of maybe as much as five or six pounds a week are no longer happening. The going is slower, less spectacular. The routine may seem boring. There may even be a perverse part of you that doesn't like the idea of your being thinner. This perverse part was buried during the initial energy outpouring, but as the energy wanes, it may begin to rear up.

This motley crew of distractions sets about seducing you into abandoning your weight control program. In order to do this, the conspirators use a very devious tactic. Never for a moment will they suggest you abandon your goal. These blackguards are far too clever for that. What they do is to insidiously create the idea that you have been so good; now you are in real control; that a little deviation for a meal, a day, or during your vacation won't hurt. You're entitled to a little treat. You can start again any time. Haven't you proved how easy this is, how good you are?

Don't Believe It! This is a most perilous time, this period following your early successes when you begin to think that it is clear sailing from here on. It is during this critical period that the true success of your weight control program will be determined. Don't slacken now! *Reach your goal!* The probability is too great that if you fall into the seductive trap you will quickly drift back into the old gain-weight syndrome. Eating things you have been avoiding can make you yearn for a lot of old taste temptations that you haven't been away from very long. Remember, it is easier not to eat the first potato chip than not to eat the second one. By abstaining from, or limiting your intake of, these fat-creating tastes, you have started developing a numbness toward them. You are beginning to lose some of the intense desire for these tastes. While it is still possible to feel deprived in your mind, your body is beginning to be freed from the intense desire for these fat producers. Abstinence works toward non-interest.

On one diet I didn't eat ice cream for a number of months. Then I started feeling badly about something and I bought a quart of ice cream and started eating it. The first portion was not that pleasurable. But after I had this first portion I kept on eating the ice cream. My body was not craving it, but my mind was pushing me, remembering how it used to feel. Within a short time I was hooked again on a real bodily craving level. The same was true of smoking the first pack of cigarettes after I had quit for five years. I didn't really like the first cigarettes, but by the second or third pack I was right back into the addiction. Once you start tasting those certain foods again, the tastes feed on themselves. You start to want more. The desire is reinforced and you are soon back to the old problem of starting all over again.

It is important to hear what I am saying in perspective. I am not saying: become a fanatic, cloister yourself, shut yourself off. I am saying: stay away from those things that trigger you. With me, it's ice cream and bread products. I know myself. You know yourself. It doesn't mean I would not take a helping of stuffing at a turkey dinner or a small piece of birthday cake at a party. The eating of such foods occasionally in moderate amounts is not going to have a real effect upon my weight. But I am not going to have a pint of ice cream and a whole pizza, both of which I am capable of doing. To eat those would dangerously seduce me away from my weight control program toward more ice cream and more pizza tomorrow. Now that I have my weight under control, I do at times have two or three pieces of pizza or a scoop of ice cream. But when I do, I am treading on dangerous ground and I must be alert to be sure to stop. I will try to eat these addictive foods slowly and drink a lot of liquids with them in order to help control the urge to continue eating them reflexively.

A second reason for not falling into the "I'll just go off it for a little while" trap is the psychology that surrounds taking a step backward. It is something like the feeling you would have if after pushing a heavy boulder half way up a mountain, you were suddenly pushed back a hundred yards by a strong wind. Having to rework the same ground is discouraging and requires summoning up even more energy than is required to keep slogging along. I'm not saying it can't be done. Of course it can. It just is self-defeating to take a step backward. It makes the job harder.

A third reason for not straying from the path is that by doing so, we lose touch with the satisfaction we can get from nonfattening tastes. This not only makes the short-term weight loss phase more difficult, it also detracts from our long-term weight maintenance program. We want to subdue, if not totally eradicate, the felt need for those fattening foods that turn us on. We want to be able to easily turn away from them whenever necessary. We do this by abstaining from the fattening foods and staying in touch with the satisfaction we can truly get from nonfattening foods. When we stop eating nonfattening foods, we lose touch with the satisfaction they offer. Also, we want the size of our appetite to diminish. Eating fattening foods or overeating now will tend to frustrate these long-term goals. Over the long term, we are creating a skill, the skill of weight control. Continued practice makes the skill stronger whereas lack of practice tends to have the opposite effect.

What you need to do to combat the insidious urge to stray for "just a little while" is to sustain the energy (the enthusiasm) that got you started. Keep in touch with your intention and motivation. Keep in touch with why you want to lose weight and the pitfalls of giving in. Keep creating the right associations in your mind. Say those things suggested in Chapters 3 and 6 before meals, when arising in the morning, and at bedtime. They will help keep the energy alive.

It may also help if you give yourself some form of shock. Shocks create energy. A shock will shake you up. Have you ever been in an automobile accident or unexpectedly tripped and fell? Didn't your body vibrate as your energy flowed like electricity? There was no appetite for food then. A self-created shock will have to be less dramatic and, of course, not a real danger. We aren't going to have auto accidents or go tripping about to shock ourselves. But we may be able to create a shock-like effect with our imaginations. For example, does any particular visual image stimulate your enthusiasm for weight control or take away your appetite? Maybe it is the image of yourself as a fat person being shunned by others. Maybe a collection of pictures of fat people (a rogues gallery) that you have clipped from magazines and newspapers will do it. I am particularly sensitive to scenes of people in operating rooms of hospitals. The vivid scene of someone being cut and bleeding, and then sewn up, will take away my appetite. Use imagery. Whatever works, use it. Don't spare yourself.

Keep in touch with how difficult it was to start. Once you let go, that difficulty will be there again. Retrigger your resolve. Remember, if you successfully deflect the urge to stray now, the urge will die, not grow, and will be less difficult and less intense in the future. It is like an athlete getting a second wind. If you go just a little farther, you get in touch with a new and even more powerful energy source. If you stray now, you can't be sure when you will start again.

The urge to stray from your weight control program may be, in part, due to boredom with the routine. Think about ways to increase the variety of what you are eating. Keep adding to your list of pleasurable nonfattening foods. Harness that energy pushing you to stray, and use it to meet the challenge by finding new, satisfying, nonfattening tastes.

When you start to think about deviating from your weight control program, it may be because you are hungry or hunger is creeping up on you. So when you consider straying, check if you are hungry, and if so, eat something nonfattening that you like. Maybe something sweet. Some food in your stomach may help do the job of keeping you on the straight and narrow. If you are not hungry, there is no legitimate reason to stray. You are succumbing to a phantom urge. Reread the chapter on the Law of Distraction. Get into something that really grabs you. Reread the chapter on the Law of Deflection. Deflect the urge to give in.

Also know that feeling light is not necessarily being light. You are feeling relatively lighter than you were and it is a good feeling. A part of the sack on your back has dropped away. But you are only truly light when you reach your realistic weight goal, your clothes fit as they should, and you look the way you would like. This relatively lighter feeling is truly a seduction that has led me astray on a number of occasions. After I had been on one of my earlier diets for a few weeks, I felt like a million dollars—a lot lighter and a lot livelier than I had been. I remember coming home late one night and going into the kitchen to eat a little something. I saw a bagel and I ate it. Why not? Wasn't I good, feeling great, in control. Then I ate a second and a third bagel, telling myself that I could stop any time. I just wanted to see if I could still eat those foods I used to crave. Well, that was the end of that diet. The way to keep the good feeling is to not be seduced into straying off the path before your goal is reached. Let the desire to continue having the good feeling help re-arouse the energy you need to keep moving forward.

You need to keep the spark that got you started alive so that it will develop into a flame that can never be extinguished. In order to do this, you need to be on guard, to recognize and resist the tempting voice of the serpent saying "You have been so good; you can start again; a little treat won't harm you. Just for a little while." But if you do choose to stray, don't punish yourself. Forget it! Just pick yourself up and get started again. Immediately, immediately—not tomorrow or Monday! Now! Just as the more quickly someone who falls off a horse gets back in the saddle, the less psychological effect the fall will have in making him or her fearful of riding, the more quickly you return to the weight control path, the more chance there is that you will be able to pick up where you left off rather than having to go through the whole sordid starting process again after regaining all the weight you lost, plus. Remember, the whole idea of weight control is to make you feel good. So if you stray, don't make yourself feel worse by staying off the path.

The following thoughts from a book by Joseph Goldstein entitled "The Experience of Insight" are wonderfully appropriate for the midpoint of the first phase (the weight loss phase) of one's weight control program. "Now is the time to arouse energy, not to slacken. Think how much you have done...a great strength has been developing, a momentum ...the beginning was laying the foundation...the practice is slowly deepening...no one can be sure when the opportunity will come again." Nobody can be sure when and if he or she will start again. Don't let the spark die.

[18]

Haste Makes Waste

THERE IS PROBABLY nothing more counterproductive to losing weight and keeping it off than the almost universal desire to shed the allotted number of pounds in the shortest period of time. This craving for speed is reflected in the claims for different diets that one frequently sees advertised on the covers of popular magazines. Claims like "Lose 10 pounds in 7 days," or "30 days to a more slender figure" are trumpeted as inducements to the overweight to buy the magazine or other periodical. Such claims may be absolutely true. But for a number of reasons, catering to the urge to get the diet over with fast almost guarantees failure along the path to effective weight control.

First, just having the idea in one's mind that "I must get this over with fast" suggests that there is an ordeal, a burden to come. I know that feeling of "I just want to get the bloody thing over with." But such a sorrowful thought process lays the foundation for failure. There is no burden in intelligent weight control. There is no sense of deprivation. It is a challenging, creative experience. It is a stimulating game that one simply has to learn to play skillfully.

Secondly, losing more than just a few pounds is going to take some time. After a splash of early success during the first week or two, when one may drop five to ten pounds, weight loss becomes a slow process of losing a small amount of weight each week (one-half pound to three pounds for an average person depending on your sex, age, lifestyle, how rigidly you are dieting, how overweight you are, and how much exercise you may or may not do). When you start thinking about how quickly you can get this over with, you are not preparing yourself for the relatively slow nature of the process. You are creating a mindset in which during a moment of frustration with the seemingly petty pace, you will be tempted into chucking the whole thing. Once you do that, you are back at square one, struggling with the problem of starting all over again as the pounds pile on.

Thirdly, and absolutely most importantly, what is the hurry? What are you racing toward? Hopefully not to the time when the ordeal will be over and you can eat again. That will only lead to a relapse into the ways that have kept us on the gain weight-diet-gain weight-diet treadmill we want to get off. What one should be looking forward to is the time that he or she won't be controlled by food and appetite but rather will be in control of them. And that time will come.

What we are trying to accomplish is not just to lose weight. If that is your only goal, most assuredly you will gain it all back again. We are learning the skill of weight control. We want to once and for all break that hideous cycle of gaining weight, dieting, gaining weight, etc. In order to do this, we need to adjust some of our responses to food. We need to create responses that will keep us off the get-fat again treadmill. And that takes a bit of time, since one must unhorse other responses acquired as a child and constantly reinforced through the intervening years. Continual repetition creates tendencies. Thus the longer we consciously remain in the initial weight loss phase of our program, the more successful we are going to be in creating and in particular reinforcing those new tendencies that will prevent us from eating in a manner that will cause us to regain the lost weight. With practice, all skills strengthen.

I reflect what I consider to be an American disposition to do things quickly. I always wanted to get a diet over with fast. I also reflect an American disposition to do things the easy way (why not?). Well, it took me years to learn that the quickest and easiest way to truly get my weight under control was to lose weight slowly. Remember the story of the tortoise and the hare. It really is true when it comes to weight control. Be the tortoise. Make haste slowly. If you are in a big hurry, you are apt to burn out like a meteor. If you move slowly, relentlessly, not paying attention to how long it is going to take, but how you feel and look, steadily moving to your goal; the chances of success are much greater. Then by the time you have reached your weight control goal, you will have created and reinforced new ways of doing things in relation to food that will make it possible for you to automatically maintain the lower weight. What makes this slow, steady pace possible is realizing that you will never be hungry, and that you are always going to have lots of good tastes.

[19]

Hide the Scale

A SYMPTOM OF the very destructive "get it over with quickly" malady discussed in the last chapter is the tendency most dieters have to weigh themselves frequently. While in the first week or two, one is often charged up by the great success the scale shows, it isn't long before the weight loss slackens to a snail's pace and one starts to feel disappointed.

In my early diets I weighed myself every day, eagerly going to the scale each morning to see my success. Of course it wasn't long before I was disappointed at my sniveling pace and truly depressed on those days when the scale inexplicably showed I actually had gained a bit. During subsequent diets, to ensure better results, I would weigh myself only once a week. Then the weekly progress also seemed insignificant, so as my weight cycled higher and the diets of necessity became longer, I went to monthly readings. Later on I moved to what I called my "National Holiday Diet." I would only weigh myself on national holidays, and not all of those, either (Thanksgiving is too close to Christmas!). The National Holiday Diet set the tone for a long battle. When in August you tell yourself that you won't set foot on the scale until Christmas, you know you are settling in for a long siege. You are setting your mind in the proper direction.

Finally, I gave up weighing myself altogether. While I

never knew exactly what I weighed, I always knew how I was doing by the way my clothes fit and what notch my belt was on. (I figured about ten pounds per notch.) When my clothes, which were always tight at the beginning of a diet, began to feel loose, I knew something important had happened. When I had to have a suit altered, something really significant had taken place.

When losing weight, I found weighing myself to be counterproductive. It is depressing to see only little bits of progress when you believe you have been so good, and feel so light, that it seems as if the weight must be melting off. It isn't! The reality is that progress is painfully slow when measured against one's efforts on a day-to-day basis. This meager progress, if dwelled upon, can too easily create frustration and a "what's the use?" attitude. One has to summon up new bursts of energy to combat the disappointingly slow pace. The progress seen in the way your clothes are fitting better or becoming too big is much more gratifying, and will provide much more positive incentive than will the slow, plodding readings of the scale. Focus attention on the readings your body and your clothes are giving, not on the scale. The number on the scale is an abstraction to carry in your mind. The fit of your clothes and the feel of your body is something real that you can see, and feel good about, every moment of every day. The real goal is not only to weigh a certain number of pounds, but to look and feel a certain way. You are getting a constant reading from your clothes and your body as to how you are doing in this regard.

There is an important side benefit that comes from focusing on your clothes and how you feel. We all need reinforcement for our accomplishments. Most frequently we don't get enough of it from a world of people who, understandably, are burdened by their own pressing concerns. You will get some oohs and ahs when you lose weight and that can be a reinforcer. But the acclaim will be sporadic and die out. The way your clothes and body feel is with you constantly, helping to reinforce your intention and helping you to remember at the critical moment of, "Now that I am hungry, what am I going to do?" why you want to control your weight, how badly you will feel if you don't choose the non-fattening way, and that there is a tasty Low Calorie Solution to your hunger.

Of course, you can weigh yourself at the beginning of the weight loss phase so that, if you wish, you can calculate how much weight you actually lose. I even stopped doing that in later diets. (I didn't really care exactly how much weight I lost. Only that I reached my goal.) And you may want to weigh yourself once a week for a week or two to assure yourself that you are losing weight. But that should be it. Stop weighing yourself. Set some goal about the way you want your clothes to fit. (I wanted to fit comfortably into size 34 slacks.) When you have reached this fit of your clothes goal, then weigh yourself. If you have lost as much weight as you set out to lose and you feel good, that's terrific. You are now ready for the next phase, the "Keeping It Off Phase" of your weight control program. If you have lost less weight than was your original goal, and you really feel that this lesser amount is sufficient, it's okay to adjust your goal upward to this higher level. But if you are not genuinely satisfied, then put the scale away and set a new clothes-fit goal (possibly another notch in a belt). If you have lost more than you thought you wanted to, or now seems prudent, you can consider whether you want to put back a few pounds. But if you do, put the weight back very gradually. This is a really dangerous process. Be very careful! No binges! A binge will undo the new eating patterns that you have established, and will probably lead both to a greater weight gain than you want and a need to summon up a new burst of energy to halt the upward spiral. You will probably have to start all over again.

While I recognize that there are occasions when there are legitimate reasons for weighing oneself, avoid doing it just for the sake of curiosity. The depressing fallout that can flow from any weighing is so potentially harmful that a weighing for curiosity's sake alone should be avoided. An excellent example of this dangerous phenomenon arose on my final diet. Fortunately I was far enough along the path to handle it, but it was a close call.

On my final diet I had set a goal for myself of 175 pounds, or fitting into size 34 slacks, whichever came first. Though I had no real idea of what I weighed when I started, I knew from the fit of my clothes I was heavier than I had ever been. I estimated that it would take me at least six months to reach my goal, and I tentatively set the day exactly six months from the day I began as the moment I would first mount the scale. After five months of keeping the low calorie faith, some of the malevolent seductions I spoke of in Chapter 17, "Midstream," began to work on me. I was beginning to feel really light, and I became concerned that I might be losing too much weight. Possibly exceeding my 175-pound goal.

So with a friend eagerly looking on I weighed myself (a month before the schedule called for). I needn't have worried about losing too much weight. I was still well above my goal, which is the upper end of the recommended range for someone my height and frame that one finds on the life insurance charts.

Now having weighed myself, I decided to indulge my curiosity further. I decided to figure out how much weight I was losing per week so that I could make a new and firmer estimate of when the losing weight portion of my weight control program would be over. I would make this calculation by weighing myself in another four weeks, first finding my total loss over the four week period and then dividing by four to find the average weekly loss. Knowing my average weekly weight loss would allow me to calculate about how many weeks it would take me to get down to my 175-pound goal.

I spent the next four weeks eagerly anticipating how much weight I would lose over the whole period. I tried to keep my imagination in bounds, thinking that maybe I would lose five pounds, but secretly hoping for ten or more. When the big day came, I weighed myself. To my horror, the scale said that I had not lost a pound! I didn't believe it. I stood transfixed looking down at the scale. I took the scale outside and weighed myself in the sunlight, hoping that I had mis-seen where the scale's arrow was pointing. I had seen correctly. I was really shaken.

To say that I was discouraged is putting it mildly. But I restrained the urge to eat something sweet, which frequently arises in me when I am feeling low. I resolved to think about what was going wrong, rather than to start eating, binging in distress. I thought about what I had been eating, counting my calories, wondering whether I was somehow miscounting. No! That wasn't it.

I knew from the fit of my clothes that doing exactly what I had been doing over the last four weeks, I had lost a lot of weight during the prior five months. I had gone from a tight size 40 slacks to a comfortable 36. I estimated I had lost about 40 pounds. But now everything seemed to have stopped.

There were only three possible explanations. The first was that (since, as one loses weight, it takes fewer calories to maintain one's weight at the reduced level), I might have gotten down to the weight level where my calorie intake was now equal to the calories of energy I was expending so that my weight would remain steady unless I cut my intake further. The second possibility was that I had hit the scale on an off day; that I had really lost a little weight which had just not shown up on that particular day. The final possibility was that the scale was broken (my favorite possibility, though the least probable).

A few days later I weighed myself again, and to my relief, I was three pounds lighter. Thus, while I had not lost as much weight as I had expected and not nearly as much as I had secretly dreamed about, at least I had not been shut out. I was going to have to accept a weight loss of less than a pound a week and it was going to still be quite some time until I reached my goal of 175 pounds—longer than I had originally thought. This was a bit distressing, but I knew there was a blessing in disguise. The longer it took to reach the goal, the more used to the program I would become, and the easier it would be when I did reach my goal to keep my weight under control. Originally I had hoped to reach my goal in six months; it took me ten. But I reached it.

Another blessing in disguise that flowed from this experience was the recognition that I had not abandoned the program in the face of the disappointment. In fact, before I weighed myself again the second time, I had made some minor adjustments in my eating routine that cut a hundred calories or so from my daily intake. I was determined to reach 175 pounds, fit comfortably into size 34 slacks, or bust. I believe that not eating in response to this disappointment, but rather trying to understand and cope with it ensured my not going back onto the gain weight-diet treadmill. Later I could also see how my positive approach to the disappointment had strengthened me in dealing with disappointments in other areas of my life. I had established a model of dealing positively with a frustrating experience that would serve me in good stead, not only in the weight control area, but elsewhere as well.

But positive as it turned out to be, this episode reinforced my belief that weighing yourself while reducing can be pretty dangerous and should be avoided unless absolutely necessary. However, while your scale is best unseen during the reducing portion of a weight control program, it isn't by any means a useless relic. As I will explain in the chapter "Keeping it Off," it will immediately regain a place in the sun as soon as you have reached a weight that completely satisfies you. But until then, it's best to forget about it.

[20]

Those Witching Hours After Dark

HOW MANY TIMES have I heard a failed dieter say something like, "I'm okay until the evening. Then everything falls apart. My diet goes up in smoke. I just pig out." Do I know what they mean! I have blown many a diet between 8:00 P.M. and midnight. The nighttime problem is one of the biggest that the successful dieter must overcome. And it is easy enough to do, once the problem is truly understood.

What happens in the evening is that we tend to unwind. We tend to relax. Most critically, our attention, which has been focused during the day on the tasks of our daily routine, often now roams around without very much to do. The focus of the day has given way to a period of unfocused activity. Frequently, we are sitting around relaxing, looking for something to do, possibly bored. When we have nothing absorbing us, our attention frequently goes toward food— and we eat.

Even though nighttime attacks can be really intense, the way to handle this nighttime problem is no different than the way to handle any attack of Phantom Hunger.

1. Use the Law of Distraction. Realize that the problem is unfocused energy, and try to absorb yourself in some activity.

2. If you eat, use the Law of Deflection. Drink lots of liquids (especially hot liquids) with whatever you are eating to further dilute the Phantom Hunger attack.

3. As always before any snack, remember to ask yourself if you are really hungry and if this is the Low Calorie Solution.

4. If you can, try to eat slowly. When we finish breakfast or lunch, we rush off to deal with the day's activity, but nighttime eating is often followed by more unfocused time. Eating slowly and diluting the hunger with hot liquids will help combat the urge to keep cramming the food in.

5. Be sure there is no addictive food in the house, or if there is, be sure it is somewhere that you can't get at it (locked up with someone else having custody of the key). At night, the danger of succumbing to an addiction is really extreme, as it is at any time when we are not focused on some activity.

Another way to handle the nighttime problem is to eat dinner late. The later you finish dinner, the less time until you go to bed. And the less time the nighttime varmint has to strike. But it isn't possible for everyone to change their dinner hour and it isn't necessary. Simply by applying the Laws of Distraction and Deflection, and doing the other things suggested, you can handle the nighttime plague in the same manner as you handle any attack of Phantom Hunger.

Another problem that can arise after dark comes from waking in the middle of the night with a feeling of Phantom Hunger. I have often awakened in the middle of the night with a throbbing energy that prevented me from going back to sleep. As indicated in Chapter 15 on emotional hunger, when one has a throbbing energy and no place to direct it, one may eat in order to try and relieve the inner tension. In the middle of the night, after tossing around in bed, unable to get back to sleep, I would go into the kitchen to raid the refrigerator and food cupboard. I would eat a lot when I wasn't even hungry. I was just looking for something to do, trying to snuff out that swirling energy that was keeping me awake.

As I became more aware of weight control and what I was doing in those middle-of-the-night eating bouts, I developed a tactic that has worked well in handling this problem. Instead of eating a lot, I would just eat a little something, maybe two or three spoons of cottage cheese or a couple of pieces of Melba Toast, to settle my stomach and help calm the energy. After such a small snack, I could get back to sleep. A light touch worked as well as a heavy hand. In fact, it worked better, because if I binged, when I awoke in the morning, I felt badly. I had an unpleasant aftertaste in my mouth and a sour stomach. But when I tread lightly, I never have those unpleasant sensations.

If you awaken in the middle of the night as I do, and feel the need to eat something, go ahead, eat, but keep it very light. Just have a touch of something. Find things to eat that are light and nonfattening that will settle you down. And be sure these items are on the list of satisfying low calorie foods that is taped to the door of your refrigerator and food cupboard.

[21]

Four Snakes in the Grass

THERE ARE FOUR SITUATIONS that often present a set of somewhat similar and intense challenges to a weight control program. These are, eating out, vacations, parties, and coffee breaks. The unique problems posed by these occasions are as follows: (1) they are often socially stressful, and many people, especially overweight people, try to relieve stress by eating—possibly even stuffing; (2) the choice of nonfattening foods tends to be limited; (3) there are a lot of tempting goodies conspiring to seduce us into eating something we will assuredly regret having eaten; and (4) the occasion is festive and we feel that we don't want to deprive ourselves at such a joyful time, especially since everybody else is living it up, or, I should say, eating it up. Let's deal with these situations, one at a time, focusing on how we can develop simple strategies that will empower us to beat back their challenge.

The problem of eating out is best handled by going to a restaurant that offers nonfattening foods you like. I usually opt for a Chinese or other Oriental restaurant where there are many dishes with rice and vegetables that I enjoy or for a health food restaurant where I can have an interesting type of salad or something else I find tasty that is relatively low in calories. Unfortunately, when with others, I don't always get my way, and I often find myself in a restaurant (probably

Italian) where the menu is much less conducive to weight control. However, even here I cope. First, I stay away from the bread and butter, which will really do me in. I get a salad in front of me as soon as possible. I may well order a second salad to help fill me up. Then I will have a pasta dish, usually with a relatively less-fattening sauce. I drink a bottle or two of beer (possibly light beer) with the salad and main course. At dessert time, I may have some tea with a low-cal sweetener (or even real sugar). I am satisfied, happy, and have survived the meal with very little damage (if any) to my weight control program.

Almost any restaurant will have something relatively low calorie, like salads, vegetables, rice, baked potatoes, fruit, fish dishes, etc., that I like and that will fill me up. Along with the filler, I might eat something else, which, though not as low calorie as I might prefer, is still not outrageous. If you think about the challenge, most restaurants will offer enough tasty, nonfattening foods to allow you to enjoy the meal and still feel good about yourself. Much better than if you allow the problem of eating out to serve as an excuse for letting up on your program.

Vacations just pose a specialized version of the eating out problem. Almost anywhere you go, you should be able to find acceptable, tasty foods that are nonfattening. What is different about the vacation situation is the idea that most of us have, that on a vacation we should live it up, and be free of any restrictions. We want to have the most fun possible. Who wants to be concerned about their weight on a vacation?

If you want to get the most out of your vacation, use it as a time to start your weight control program—not as an excuse to gain weight. You will feel much better when you come home if you have lost a few pounds rather than gaining five or ten that you will have to cope with for a lot longer than the week or two you were on vacation. The idea that a vacation is not a time to start a weight control program, or even worse, that it is a time to suspend one (which almost always means the end of the program), arises from the mistaken notion that controlling one's weight must be an ordeal. It doesn't have to be! It can be a stimulating, challenging game. On your vacation, look for new low calorie, satisfying foods. Maybe back home they are in the foreign food, gourmet or regular sections of your grocery store and thus available to continue enhancing your weight management program.

Of course, if there is a local dish which you really can't find at home, or a local five star restaurant with a specialty that can't be duplicated, a once-in-a-lifetime opportunity, or even a once-in-a-year experience, go ahead; enjoy it, and don't feel guilty. It won't wreck your weight control program unless you allow the event to be an excuse to indulge yourself in things that are not unique, and will just pile on the pounds. The pleasant experience will soon fade, but a weight problem is going to present you with a lot of continuous not-so-pleasant experiences.

A party presents varying problems, depending on the degree of social stress involved, what is being served, and how well you know the host or hostess. The easiest solution is to simply find the veggies and keep munching them (possibly with a little dip). But if there are no veggies or similar low calorie foods, you need to do something to keep yourself comfortable, especially if you are going to be at the party for a while. Remember, liquids fill. Look for plain and diet sodas. I also (as discreetly as possible) suck the ice, which helps keep something trickling into my stomach, and keeps my mouth busy in a fashion that is akin to what it would be doing if I were eating. In addition, the ice numbs my taste buds, and this helps kill the urge for food. And I suspect that sucking the ice may help relieve my stress much in the way that sucking my thumb did when I was a little kid!

Don't nibble anything you are addicted to. If you know the host or hostess well enough, or even if you don't, meander into the kitchen and see if you can find something appropriate in the refrigerator or elsewhere. I do this frequently. If somebody chances by, don't be shy. Tell them what your problem is. You will probably get a lot of sympathy and possibly a good idea.

However, if you prefer not to be skulking around someone

else's kitchen hunting for nonfattening foods, there are two, possibly three, other ways to handle the eating-at-a-party problem. The first I learned from Scarlett O'Hara's nanny in "Gone With the Wind." Scarlett's nanny would always cram Scarlett full of food before sending her off to a party so that at the gala, Scarlett would be a proper, dainty, Southern belle with the appetite of a sparrow. Well, you and I can do the same thing before going to a party. We can eat a lot so we are full and don't have any Real Hunger. The second idea is to take something along to eat at the party, possibly a piece of fruit in a pocket or purse. The third way that I have used to handle the party problem is only available if you are near a built-up shopping area. Go out to a nearby grocery store or coffee shop, and have something to eat. Then come back. You probably won't be missed. I almost never am.

The last viper in the grass, the coffee break, is really best handled by observing the Boy Scout motto, "Be Prepared." Bring something from home to eat during the coffee break. I will almost always bring a piece of fruit. The fruit will give me the same sweet taste that others are experiencing in eating pastries, etc., but I stay slim while they are piling on the pounds.

Thus, while eating out, vacations, parties, and coffee breaks may require some planning ahead, imagination, or flexibility, they are not difficult to handle. All you need is the intention not to be trapped into giving in and the satisfying Low Calorie Solution will appear. It's Always There!

[22]

Keeping It Off

THE GREATEST PROBLEM most people have in controlling their weight is not losing pounds, but rather keeping them off—what many call "maintenance." Losing weight just to gain it all back-plus, then lose it and gain it again, is not only ridiculous, it is unhealthy and unnecessary. But that is exactly what I did for years, and what all people who are struggling with their weight are doing.

This problem arises because the dieter, sometimes after reaching his or her goal, but usually before, slips back into the destructive patterns that caused his or her gaining weight in the first place. This book is explaining an effective way to cope with, to get around, these patterns. When you cope with them successfully for a long enough period, they will fade away completely. But that takes time. A long time! A lot more time than the weight loss period. It was not until years after I stopped smoking that I truly did not find myself enjoying the smell of smoke. While when I was not exposed to the smell of smoke I never felt any desire, once I got a few whiffs of the aroma of a lit cigarette, the urge came to life. So it is with fattening foods. We have now eliminated our need for them and found equal satisfaction elsewhere. But if we over-expose ourselves to these temptations, they will once again hook us. We are not enslaved any more. But we are not yet truly free. We are winning the battle. But the enemy is not completely routed. It is still a threat. This is the reality, and we must accept it or else stay on the treadmill. During the weight loss phase of the program you have learned to cope with the destructive patterns effectively. But you have not blown them to kingdom come.

The "Keeping It Off" phase of your weight control program should just flow smoothly out of the "Taking It Off" phase. Nothing really changes. It is crucial to understand that we have not been on a diet. We have been learning and practicing the skill of weight control. This is just another stage, a natural growth of our weight control program. There is no fanfare ushering us into a new period of license to be heedlessly sinful. This is not the beginning of "Thank God, it's over. Now I can eat again." By always eating when you were hungry, and by learning to find low calorie foods that you enjoy during the weight loss period, you have eliminated any sense of deprivation. Just the realization that there are lots of low calorie foods that taste good to you makes the maintenance phase easy and automatic.

Eating isn't going to be substantially more enjoyable now, because it never became substantially less enjoyable. You are entitled to feel good about your success. Feel good! Feel great! But the game is not over. You are just beginning a new phase.

After reaching your goal, you flow into the "Keeping It Off" phase by adding calories to your self-tailored plan. Raise your daily calorie count to the amount needed to keep your weight stable. You will probably have to experiment a bit to find what this daily maintenance rate should be. Add the calories back a little at a time. At first, add 200 calories to your daily average. After a week, see what effect these extra calories have had on your weight. If you are still losing, add another 200 calories to your daily average, and after another week see what has happened. When you stop losing, you have reached the daily average that will keep your weight at its current level.

Although you have reached your goal, you must continue doing some of the things you did in the "Taking It Off" phase of the program. It is essential to *continue counting calories* each day. This continuing focus on your calorie intake will be the single most important factor ensuring success in the maintenance phase of your weight control program. It is also essential to stay conscious of your weight control program by always remembering to say at the beginning of every meal and before every snack those things we have been saying: why we want to control our weight; how badly we will feel if we overeat; and to remember to choose the low calorie solution. And, it is very important to continue *using your list,* and adding to it new low calorie foods, food combinations and recipes that you find tasty.

Also, as much as possible, one needs to shy away from addictive foods. When you eat them, do it very carefully, very slowly, and at the same time, drink plenty of low calorie liquids.

Finally, keep this book in a place where you can see it. Seeing this book will help you hear my voice talking to you, saluting you, saying, "Good show! Keep up the good work! Remember why you want to control your weight; how much better you will feel if you stay at this weight instead of letting yourself go; that there is always a Low Calorie Solution available."

The reason why many successful dieters, who have reached their weight loss goal, who feel a great resolve never to gain the weight back, and who even may keep the pounds off for a while eventually drift back onto the gain weight treadmill is that their resolution ebbs as their energy is distracted by other pursuits. They do not realize that the victory is not complete and they do not have a plan to mop up the remaining pockets of enemy resistance.

The way to harness the energy needed to maintain our weight is to keep popping weight control back into our consciousness. We do this by continuing to count calories, to say those things we have learned to say before meals and snacks, and to keep our list of low calorie foods updated and ever available. These actions keep our minds focused on weight control and this focus keeps our energy channeled properly.

The successful dieter who falls back into the abyss has no plan to keep his or her energy channeled toward weight control. Follow the plan I am outlining and you will keep the weight off just as effortlessly and naturally as you took it off. Eventually, after we have avoided our destructive patterns long enough, they will fade into oblivion, and be replaced by more positive ones. Then we won't need the continuing reminders. Eventually, but not yet. I am certainly not at that place yet, and I am not sure when I will be.

There is one major variation in the routine of the "Keeping It Off" phase of our weight control program from the routine we followed in the "Taking It Off" phase. Now we must *weigh ourselves regularly.* Every day is okay. Once a week is a bare minimum. If you get to more than three pounds above your weight goal, *immediately* lower your daily average calorie intake back down to the amount you were eating in the "Take It Off" phase. This very moment! Now! Not tomorrow! This immediate action is crucial. You must nip the weight gain in the bud, before it really becomes a problem. Keep the "Take It Off" phase in place for one complete week. Then weigh yourself again. (Don't weigh yourself during the week.) You will probably be back at your goal. If you have not reached your goal, then continue the "Take It Off" routine for another week.

Reach your goal again! Don't just come close! Be strict with yourself and get back to your goal. The reason for this strictness, this insistence on actually reaching your goal again (even though normally during the maintenance period a fluctuation of up to three pounds from your goal is not a cause for action), is that the greater weight gain shows a tendency toward laxness, and you must quickly re-establish the proper awareness and consciousness. While a couple of pounds fluctuation in one's weight on a day-to-day basis is normal, once that fluctuation exceeds three pounds you are in a danger zone. You must act to nip the thing in the bud and prevent the laxity from becoming an incredibly large problem. You are beginning to forget. You need to jog your memory. The best way to arouse consciousness about weight control is to spend some time actively engaged in taking off weight.

If you balk at the idea of returning to the "Taking It Off" phase, as you very well may, just ask yourself if you would rather do it for a week now or for three weeks or three months later when the problem becomes worse, as it is absolutely certain to become. Make yourself answer the question. You have taken off a lot more than three pounds. It wasn't difficult. Besides asking and answering the question, also immediately start reading this book. Read the whole thing. It will stimulate the mindset you need to cope with the problem. It will help re-arouse the energy you need to meet the challenge. Remember that what you need to do is arouse energy to deal with the new weight problem. And the energy is there waiting to be roused.

You truly don't want to gain weight again. Asking and answering the question, "Would I rather do it for a week now or for three months later?" and rereading this book will help provide the shock you need to get the energy flowing. Understanding that all you need do is develop a point of view you already have, and to arouse energy that is within you, waiting to be aroused, will set you on the path of quickly acting to prevent yourself from once again putting on those pounds that will make you feel and look rotten.

As with everything else I am talking about, the "Keeping It Off" phase of the skill of weight control may take a while to completely master. But once you have consciously acted to keep the weight off, by doing what I am suggesting, you will find it happening more naturally. If you found that losing weight made you feel good, you will be elated when, after a while, you find that you can keep your weight within a three-pound range, and still be enjoying life as much, if not a lot more, than when you were piling on the pounds. It may take a couple of episodes of returning to the weight loss phase before keeping your weight under the three-pound alarm point just happens. But once you have a successful episode or two of nipping any laxity in the bud, it will be a lot easier to nip any future laxity before it gets out of hand.

Your own successful experience in keeping the weight off will serve as a model, making it easier for you to continue keeping it off. With practice, any skill becomes more and more automatic.

Understanding that you need to keep some of your energy channeled toward weight control, and having a plan to do this, is what will empower you to do what you have never done before; keep the weight off! Then you can go on and deal effectively with other challenges in your life.

[23]

My List

THE FOLLOWING ARE some of the things that I have learned to do through the years in order to handle my hunger in a nonfattening way. Some of my solutions may seem bizarre to you, possibly even unpalatable. That's fine! Remember, weight control is a very personal thing, and must be founded upon one's own unique tastes. Find your own bizarre, and possibly to me, unpalatable solutions. But try some of my ideas unless they are truly offensive, and give them a chance to work.

The granddaddy of all my solutions is to drink liquids. Hot liquids in particular, but even cold ones, especially when carbonated, are very filling. I can't stress too strongly the value of this tactic. Hot coffee, tea, or bouillon, and cold diet or plain sodas are almost calorieless ways to satisfy Phantom Hunger. They will often even temporarily sedate Real Hunger. Thus, when I feel hungry between meals, I will first have a cup of hot tea or a cold diet soda. Before I went on the coffee wagon, I used black coffee as my primary weapon against Phantom Hunger. For many years, black coffee was a mainstay of my dieting regimen. Sometimes I would add a sugar substitute such as Sweet & Low to the coffee. While I never put milk or cream in my coffee even when I wasn't dieting, if one only drinks coffee with milk, it is perfectly okay to put low fat or skim milk in the coffee. It is much better to take in a few extra calories (even a number of times during the day) than to succumb to an eating binge. You never need be fanatical about weight control. You need to use common sense. If coffee with milk will do the job of satisfying hunger, then by all means add milk.

Hot liquids tend to be a better filler than cold ones because the warmth lulls the stomach into thinking it is getting something hearty, as it often does when we eat hot foods. The first time I got in touch with the filling effect of soup was in a Real Hunger, but nondieting situation. During a summer vacation from college, a friend and I were working on a construction gang in Yellowstone Park. We had just gotten the job, and we had signed up to eat lunches in the field kitchen at the construction site. We hadn't been eating too well because we didn't have much money left from our last job. That's the kind of summer it was. When it was finally lunchtime on our first day on the new job, I was really hungry. The first thing placed on the table was a huge tureen of soup. As I was reaching for the ladle, my friend grabbed my arm, and said, "Jon, don't eat the soup. It's a filler. You want to eat solid food and get your money's worth." My friend was right. Soup is, in fact, a filler. I find that beginning a meal with, or eating as a snack, bouillon, consomme; or even a more hearty soup that is relatively low in calories, such as tomato, vegetable, or Manhattan (red) clam chowder, is an excellent way to subdue an urge to eat.

Frequently, instead of a hot liquid, I will drink a diet or a plain soda. (I am aware that diet sodas are not sound nutritionally and suspect healthwise. I will work on eliminating them someday, but for now, they are useful in helping me with what I feel is a more basic problem, keeping my weight under control.) Besides offering the filling effect that any liquid will, a carbonated beverage, because of its gasiness, creates an increased feeling of fullness. I think that the satisfying effect of foods high in fiber, at least in part, may come from the fact that they create a certain amount of gasiness. At least, they do in me.

If the liquid alone can't satisfy my hunger, I will often have it in combination with some solid food such as an apple, a salad, or a raw vegetable such as celery, carrots, cucumbers or cherry tomatoes. I consider any of these to be very satisfying low calorie snacks when I am *really* hungry. The combination of the liquid and one of these foods will usually satisfy any attack of between meal hunger I experience.

A second idea of value is that chewy foods tend to give more satisfaction for less calories than do smooth foods. It takes time and effort to eat chewy things, while smooth foods just slide down quickly, inviting you to stuff more in. If you chew a lot, it is work. One gets tired of chewing, and this will affect the desire to eat more. A good example of this idea in action is when I compare the effect of snacking on an apple rather than a scoop of ice cream. I find that I very rarely can eat a second apple while I can always have more ice cream.

A third very basic solution to my hunger problems came from learning to accept the use of a small amount of a high calorie taste enhancer as a way to get me to eat a much larger quantity of a low calorie food than I would have enjoyably eaten otherwise. I don't hesitate to use a small quantity of something I like that may be relatively high in calories to create desirable tastes. But I am very careful; very, very careful; not to douse the low calorie food that I am eating with the higher calorie goodie.

A favorite food combination of mine used to be lettuce and ketchup. (I used to be a ketchup freak—so much so that a next-door neighbor once gave me a case of ketchup as a birthday present.) But since I have now stopped eating ketchup, I have to forgo this tasty combination. I do use dips with veggies, sour cream on potatoes, and dressings on salads. I just don't use very much of the high calorie combining food. This idea of adding just a touch of a higher calorie enhancer to a low calorie food can be extended as far as your imagination and taste buds will take you, but always should be done quite carefully.

Before leaving this idea of using combining foods to make low calorie things taste good, I want to mention herbs and spices. While I have never learned to do it, it seems clear to me that coming to understand which herbs and spices one likes and then using them in combination with low calorie foods as "flavor enhancers" will be a big assist in weight control.

My favorite low calorie nighttime and between-meal snacks, besides those mentioned earlier, include popcorn, an orange, cottage cheese with diet jam (or even a small amount of regular jam), and celery with a small amount of cottage or ricotta cheese. Other favorite snacks I rely on are a big piece of honeydew melon, cantaloupe, or watermelon, some grapes, or a dish of cut-up fresh fruit. Sometimes I have a low calorie canned fruit, possibly with a couple of spoons of Cool Whip on top, which, if you stretch your imagination beyond the breaking point, you might call a diet sundae. At one time, I was eating a low calorie chocolate syrup with the Cool Whip and fruit. Unfortunately, this syrup (other people who tasted it feel with good reason) seems to have disappeared from the market. If I feel like something crunchy, I will reach for a couple of pieces of Melba Toast or a rice cake or two, which I may eat with cottage cheese or diet jam.

Another snack I find satisfying is a few large leaves of lettuce with a thin slice or two of a cheese or meat in between; in effect making a sandwich. I eat plain yogurt, sometimes with half a banana mixed in. I have also eaten frozen dietary desserts, soft frozen yogurt made with no fat milk and a frozen yogurt bar which is very satisfying and contains only 37 calories.

Whenever I am hungry between meals, or at night, I remember to eat one of these foods. They are very satisfying to me and, even eaten in relatively large quantities, offer a nonfattening way to subdue my hunger. I also remember that the hunger-satisfying value of any of these snacks is greatly magnified by drinking a hot or cold liquid.

For meals I eat some proteins and a lot of cereals, salads, vegetables and fruits. I try to minimize but not completely eliminate fats. Breakfast may be two poached eggs and two pieces of dry toast, or a bowl of oatmeal or dry cereal with non fat milk. Alternatively, breakfast might be three pancakes without butter or syrup. For lunch I will most often have a salad, usually without dressing. I always order the dressing on the side and these days almost always let it sit there. (Having the dressing available is just another security blanket.) It's there if I need it, but now I almost never do. In the past, when dieting, I always had *small* amounts of dressing with huge salads.

I often go to salad bars where I have found that a little Jell-O creates a combination, with lettuce, cucumbers, tomatoes, and mushrooms, that is every bit as satisfying to me as is salad dressing. To this combination I add a small amount of chopped eggs and chopped cheese. And of course I always avoid the salad bar items that have mayonnaise or other dressings mixed in.

When alone for dinner, I may again visit a salad bar or I may have meat, baked potato, vegetable, and a small salad. Sometimes I will have Chinese food, such as vegetable chow mein or mushi pork, with a lot of rice. I also eat pasta but without heavy, fattening sauces. Or I may just have a large bowl of cereal or rice, with a can of tuna fish packed in water, followed by a low calorie dessert.

About half of each week I eat dinner alone. I don't like to cook so I either go out or make something very simple for myself. On the other three or four nights a week I eat with a close friend, who is a very good cook and enjoys cooking. My friend usually makes vegetable, grain, poultry, or pasta-based dishes with soups, salads and fruits. She is able to enhance the flavor of foods in a very satisfying, and, when she wants to, a nonfattening manner. It is much easier for someone who enjoys cooking to make food satisfyingly tasty in a nonfattening way than it is for someone like me, who would rather go to a restaurant than boil water, and who, when he stays home, just opens packages and cans. But I make it work my way. Just as you can make it work your way.

After looking at what I eat, especially the combinations (lettuce and ketchup) or lack of them (pancakes without syrup or butter), you may be saying to yourself, "That doesn't sound bad," which it isn't; in fact, it's quite good. Or alternatively you may be saying, "I could never do that. He must be crazy." It doesn't matter. You don't have to use any of the things that I use. Just learn which low calorie foods and food combinations work for you.

Remember that all tastes are acquired. Experiment! Don't be inflexible. There was a time, not so long ago, when I wouldn't consider using fat-free milk, known as skim milk, or, to its most ardent detractors, as "blue milk." Then, after I had lost about sixty pounds on my "Final Diet," it struck me that if I used skim milk instead of low-fat milk on the plentiful quantity of cereal I was eating, not only would I receive the health benefits of eating less fat, I would also be saving on the average of a hundred calories a day. So with much trepidation and prepared for the worst, I bought a quart of skim milk and tried it on a bowl of cereal. For the first couple of bowls, I could tell the difference, but it wasn't so bad. By the time I finished the container I was feeling quite comfortable with the fat-free milk. Six weeks later, when because there was no skim milk in the house, I again used low-fat milk, it seemed like I was using cream. I could not go back to the richer low-fat milk without reconditioning myself. A similar thing happened twenty-five years earlier when I began drinking low calorie sodas. After a short time I found regular soft drinks too sweet and unpleasant tasting.

I used to hate yogurt, really hate it! But now I have developed a liking for plain, unflavored yogurt. I never ate mangoes. As a kid, one winter when I was in Florida with my family, I developed a terrible case of asthma. The doctors had no idea what was causing the illness. My mother, heaven knows why, decided that I was allergic to the mangoes that grew in Florida, and that they were causing my asthma. With this kind of introduction you can see why I never ate mangoes. Then a few years ago, a friend kept placing them on the table. I finally tried one. At first I didn't like the taste; now I do. The same is true of kiwis. At first I didn't like them; now I do.

New tastes are acquired. Old tastes change. I used to eat ketchup on everything. Now I never eat it. In earlier years, I ate hamburgers incessantly. Now, while I still eat hamburgers, I do so infrequently. I knew something had changed in my life when one day at lunch in a restaurant, I decided to have an avocado stuffed with shrimp, rather than my old standby, the hamburger. In the old days I would never have eaten an avocado. Today, I love artichokes. The first few times I tasted artichokes they seemed strange. Now I love them. My point is that if you have the intention to control your weight, you will find lots of low calorie tastes, new ones and old ones, that are satisfying to you. You can develop new tastes by exposing yourself to new things. But you need to tell your mind to start dealing with the problem, and you do that by compiling your own list, and by trying new things.

[24]

Using the Grocery Store

IF YOU AIN'T GOT IT, YOU CAN'T EAT IT. Don't buy fattening foods. Always have acceptably tasty, nonfattening foods available, but as much as possible, don't bring any of those fattening temptations that will torment you into the house. It is much easier to deal with a moment of weakness if you don't have readily available a food, that if eaten, could well spell the beginning of the end for your whole plan. A moment of weakness that you deal with successfully will help strengthen your resolve, and build the foundation of success and awareness that will empower you to deal with future moments of temptation. There will be fewer and fewer moments of weakness as your program matures, but they will still recur for a long time. If you are going to falter in some late-night binge, or at any other time, *make it difficult for yourself.* Make it so you have to get out of the house and go to a store, restaurant, or whatever. Then maybe in the time it takes you to get to the place where you can buy the sinful item you crave, your memory will have been stimulated to remind you why you want to lose weight and keep it off; how badly you will feel psychologically, emotionally and physically soon after you eat whatever it is that you are after; and what an acceptable alternative would be. Then you can still turn around, go back, and eat that alternative, which should be in your kitchen.

Time is an ally in a moment of weakness. The longer you hold off, the greater the chance that the right idea, the right feeling, the right memory will intervene and lead you to an acceptable, rather than a self-defeating solution to the momentary hunger urge. And the longer you hold off, the less intense the craving may become. You may not want the thing any more.

If you are living with others, there may be some conflicts of interest in keeping your house free of foods that can sabotage you. But try and keep as much out of the house as possible. Let the kids get their treats outside the house. Ask your spouse, other family members, or other living companions to support you in your efforts by keeping the house free of disruptive foods. Since, in controlling your weight, you will be eating a lot of nourishing, healthy foods, you may well be doing them a favor (though unfortunately, they may not see it that way). However, especially if you have growing children, there may be no reasonable way to keep the house free of everything that might do you in. In that event, segregate any of the danger foods in a separate closet, separate freezer, or separate refrigerator if these options are practical. Lock the storage place and give the key to someone else. If this is not practical, segregate the danger items in the back or in a separate section of your cupboard, freezer, or refrigerator, as much out of view as possible. The first goal is to keep as much of the addictive foods as you can out of the house. The second goal is to make whatever must slip in as inconspicuous as possible.

You can give your weight program some very positive impetus in the grocery store, not only by refraining from buying addictive foods, but also by using the time spent rolling your cart down the aisles to think about weight control. Keep looking for new ideas. Read labels to see what the calorie count of foods that interest you may be. Look for intriguing recipes on the labels of low calorie food packages. Look for new additions in the diet section. Browse through the magazines offering diet ideas and recipes for nonfattening dishes. Take some extra time in the store. An occasional good idea is worth a lot of time sleuthing about the super-market. At the very least you will have spent this time think-ing constructively about your weight control program. This thinking alone, by keeping your awareness focusing on weight control, will strengthen your intention, and contrib-ute to your being in a state of mind when hunger strikes which will guide you to the Low Calorie Solution. The re-peated attention that you give to your weight control pro-gram, and the repeated thinking about low calorie foods you like to eat, will tend to make nonfattening solutions pop into your mind at the critical moment of "Now that I am hungry, what am I going to do?"

This time in the grocery store is like a period of medita-tion about your weight control program. And like medita-tion or self-hypnosis, it will help you program your mind to make you react as you want to react. The trigger to be-ginning this meditation is truly automatic. By going into the grocery store, our minds are directed to thoughts of food. Thus, once you give your mind the signal that you want it to do it, this whole process of thinking about weight control and ways to make it more fun and more suc-cessful will be activated simply by being in the grocery store and around food.

One final and essential point is that you should never be hungry during this time in the grocery store. The fuller you are, the better. If you are hungry, the multiplicity of tempta-tions may overpower your resolve, and lead you into buying and eating things you should not. If you feel hungry when you begin shopping, immediately buy a piece of fruit or any-thing else you like that is nonfattening, possibly along with a plain or diet soda. Eat or drink what you have bought while you shop or even before you begin. Your whole being will be much more disposed toward thinking about weight control if you are satisfied and not at all hungry.

Remember, at the grocery store: don't buy fattening foods that will tempt you in moments of weakness; use the time when shopping to think about ways to enhance your weight control program; don't shop when hungry; if necessary, buy something and eat it while you are in the store. You will make your weight control program a lot easier if you will diligently follow these three suggestions.

[25]

Exercise Is Unnecessary But Helps

I HATE TO DO EXERCISE. I mean I really hate to do exercise. The thought of getting down on the floor and doing sit-ups or pushups, or otherwise bending and jumping while flailing my arms every which way, is totally repugnant to me. It may be okay for other people. But I won't do it. And nobody can make me.

When I first moved to California from upstate New York, it seemed to me as if everybody was jogging. For my part, I thought that jogging was crazy. The idea of running nowhere in particular, simply to run, seemed absolutely absurd. It seemed to me that the only reasons to run that made any sense were to get away from somewhere fast, or to have a race.

Then after I had been in California for about three years, while walking along the beach, on a beautiful, sun-drenched day, the strangest thing happened. I don't have the foggiest idea of what got into me, but just like that, I started to run. And I really enjoyed it. So much so that I started to go out to run in the morning just like all those other crazy people. Because I was woefully out of shape, and I wanted to be prudent, I started very cautiously. About 150 slow jogging steps at a time. Then a little walking. Then another 150 steps of slow jogging, more walking, and so on. But because I was a man who was always in a hurry, within a week and a half, I was jogging about two miles continuously each day, and dreaming about running marathons. However, by the end of the second week, my lurid physical past, and my overweight condition caught up with me. I developed a raft of pains throughout my body. I was sure I had done some irreparable damage.

After a series of tests, including a cardiac stress examination, it was determined, to my great relief, that there was nothing wrong with my heart. My chest discomfort, my principal concern, was probably gas-related. But I also found out that running was not very good for my back, knees, and various other parts of my anatomy, which accounted for most of my other symptoms. Though the doctor said, on balance, running would do me a lot more good than harm, I decided that my two-week running career, which had started with such promise, and engendered such wonderful dreams, was at an end. I returned to my sedentary life.

Then one morning as I lay prone on my bed watching the "Today Show" on television, I heard an interviewee talking about the glories of walking. He told how walking briskly had all the benefits of running, without the wear and tear to one's joints and vertebrae, etc. I found the information interesting, but not interesting enough to do anything about it. I filed it in the back of my mind and kept watching television.

Let me hasten to add that I have not spent all my life in such sedentary sloth, just almost all my life since I was about twenty-one. My one real flirtation with physical movement unrelated to necessary walking to my car, the refrigerator, or my desk, was a bout of bicycle riding. For a couple of years, I rode a ten-speed bicycle, possibly on the average of about twice a month. I stopped when I realized that after any extended riding, I would be very stiff and often in pain for the next day or two. I have also made a few totally unsuccessful forays onto tennis courts, golf courses, and ski slopes. After twenty-five years of periodically indulging in each of these activities (average once a year), I have neither any great passion for, nor any skill whatsoever at any of them. If I cheat, I shoot about 120 in golf, usually can't keep the ball in play at tennis, and am really not much beyond the beginner slopes in skiing. With neither pride nor embarrassment, but with a bit of disbelief that I have done so little exercise, I tell you that you now have a fairly complete picture of my lifetime physical fitness program.

Many years after my last bike ride and four years after my running career had fizzled so abruptly, with age taking its toll, my physical condition was really bleak. To put it bluntly, I was a mess. I would have to stop three times, panting breathlessly, if I happened to chance walking up a very modest grade less than half a mile long that runs in front of my house. I was afraid that the effort was putting too much stress on my heart. However, prodded as always by the fact that I was feeling lousy, and remembering that walking was supposed to be good for you, I started to go out of the house for occasional, very short walks. Nothing adventuresome. Nice, short walks. Nothing concentrated. Maybe once or twice a week. Usually on weekends.

What do you know? I liked the feeling walking gave me. I began walking more often and for longer periods of time. I started really wanting to do it. I was actually looking forward to walking. If a day went by and I wasn't able to walk, I missed it. I began walking in the area near my house, which despite a few modest grades, is fairly flat. Soon I was walking three miles a day outside the house and looking for different and more challenging walks on weekends. I started to walk up hills. I was walking every day that I could, not because I felt like I had to, but because I wanted to. If someone had told me three months before that I would voluntarily be walking every day, looking forward to it, loving it, I would have told the person that he or she was crazy. I still hate exercise, but I love walking—just as some people love running, golf, tennis, skiing, etc.

I find that walking does many good things for me. I think that any other physical activity would have the same effects. First, it is calming. It allows me to work off a lot of nervous energy that would have to be suppressed or worked off in some other way (possibly in overeating). I find getting tired physically to be very relaxing. I remember that as a student I would always study better when I was physically tired after playing some sport. When we physically exert ourselves, our nervous energy gets used up and the body feels tired, but also peaceful. I think that it is this calming feature of walking that is most appealing to me.

An interesting phenomenon about walking briskly is that as well as calming me, if I feel listless, it will also invigorate me. While the idea that something can be both calming and invigorating may seem like a contradiction, this in fact is the case. It is something akin to a grammatical oxymoron, in which a phrase like "Make haste slowly" seems to contradict itself; but in fact, the phrase is an accurate expression of a particular circumstance. While walking can calm me when my energy is high, it also can invigorate me when my energy is low. In pepping me up when I am listless, walking is turning outward energy that at the moment is directed inward and having a negative effect on how I feel.

A second benefit is that after walking briskly, my appetite is diminished. Try any brisk physical activity and see if I am not right. Remember, the exercise has to be relatively strenuous for your current physical state. Strenuous physical exercise is an appetite suppressant. Light exercise is not. In fact, light exercise may even enhance one's appetite: "Let's work up an appetite." Heavy physical exercise has the opposite effect. But before doing any strenuous exercise, be sure to check with your doctor for his approval and suggestions.

A third plus of exercise is that it burns off calories. While exercise really doesn't use up all that many calories, certainly not as many as we feel it should when we are exerting ourselves, if you exercise consistently, it adds up. For example, all other things being equal, if you use only a hundred calories each day in exercise, at the end of one year, you will weigh approximately ten pounds less than you would have if you hadn't done the daily exercise. If your daily exercise uses two hundred calories a day, you would weigh twenty pounds less at the end of a year. That is additional weight lost beyond what you may be losing as a result of limiting your calorie intake to less than you are otherwise burning in your daily routine. A chart showing the approximate number of calories of energy expended in various exercises appears in Appendix C.

Fourth, some authorities claim that exercise aids weight loss because it increases the rate at which the body burns calories, and because it builds muscle tissue that requires more calories to maintain than does body fat. Some people even claim that exercise speeds the passage of food through the body so that less calories are absorbed into the system. I pass this fourth point along without comment. I don't know if any of it is true. But if so, so much the better!

Whenever possible, I walk in the early evening before dinner. The advantage of this time is that the brisk walking acts to subdue my appetite for dinner and minimizes my nighttime snacking problem. It also helps me feel calmer and more relaxed in the evening than I would be if I had not walked off some of my nervous energy. But if I can't walk in the early evening, then I will walk anytime I can fit it in. The benefits are just as real any time of the day.

There seem to me to be a number of advantages in selecting walking as one's exercise. It is so very easy to regulate the strenuousness of the activity, just by walking faster, farther, uphill, or by doing the opposite. One can walk anywhere, and at any time. You can walk by yourself or with someone else. Since it takes no time to get ready, no major planning is needed. There is nothing to learn. There is usually no special equipment necessary, though depending upon the terrain, hiking boots or walking shoes are sometimes desirable, or even necessary.

A last attraction of walking is that it gives me a period of time alone with myself, away from the myriad of uncontrollable distractions that always seem to be intruding on me. It is a time when I do some of my clearest, and occasionally my most creative thinking. I don't plan it that way. It just happens. And not all the time! But often when I walk, something that has been troubling me pops into my head and starts to sort itself out, or I get an idea that I want to pursue.

But while walking is my favorite, it may not be yours. Any activity that you do in a relatively brisk manner for your state of physical being will offer the benefits of relaxing you, subduing your appetite, and burning off some calories.

This book is not about exercise. It is about losing weight. You don't have to exercise to lose weight. But it really helps! If you are not into some type of physical activity already, I'll bet if you really look with an open mind, you will find one you like. Frequent exercise will make controlling your weight easier and will make you feel even better. And it will probably help you to stay healthier.

Talking about health, I want to repeat this caution. Before you start any exercise program, you should discuss it with your doctor to see if she or he has any suggestion or caution to offer. "An ounce of prevention is worth a pound of cure."

[26]

About Diets

DIETS DON'T WORK! The dieter makes them work.
There are no miracle diets. When a diet succeeds, the
dieter is the miracle. It is self-defeating to think that a diet is
going to do the job for you, because such thinking distracts
attention from the fact that successful weight control requires the dieter's own *creative participation.*

Any weight loss diet is simply a food intake plan that
works because in following the plan, the dieter is eating less
calories on average each day than he or she burns. From the
viewpoint of weight control (but certainly not from the
viewpoint of nutrition), it doesn't matter if this low calorie
plan comes in the form of lots of protein, low carbohydrates, mostly fiber, pineapple and cottage cheese, or what
have you. Any plan that has you eating less calories than you
burn will ensure your losing weight, but in order to keep the
weight off, you must internalize (make a habit out of) the
discipline. And your body is not going to internalize a discipline of ultra-high protein, ultra-low carbohydrates, or any
other extraordinary eating plan dictated from outside yourself. Most of the quick weight loss diets are really alien to
our systems. What we can internalize is a *self-tailored* food
intake plan, in which we consciously choose nonfattening
foods that we like.

The odds are overwhelming that you will quit any diet

you have not created yourself in accordance with your own tastes, and return to your old fattening patterns. These old patterns are you, and all you have to fall back on. When you create your own diet to suit your own tastes, the food plan is coming from within. When you tailor-make your own diet, it isn't going to end. It is internalized already. You are recognizing certain things about tastes that you really like which will, in a nonfattening way, satisfy your hunger urges. Then when you have reached your weight goal, you will be able to add calories and expand your menu, but your weight control program will always be there with you. This is what is going to make the difference: recognizing that you are not on a diet, but mastering a skill—the skill of weight control.

If you have some allegiance to a particular diet, and it will help you get started with the weight loss phase of your program, go ahead and use it for as long as it works. But keep rereading this book so that when the enthusiasm for the diet wanes, you will begin to utilize the principles being outlined. Because unless you start to use these principles, all the pounds you have struggled to get rid of on the diet are going to come right back—plus.

Most popular diets are geared to selling you on their ability to help you lose weight quickly. And as explained in Chapter 18, "Haste Makes Waste," that point of view will ensure your quickly gaining back any weight lost. Most popular diets are fads that don't attack the problem. They are illusions, momentary palliatives, which the dieter quickly tires of paying allegiance to.

It is also possible that a diet club or a peer support group could help some people get started. The leading diet club is Weight Watchers, and the leading peer support group is Overeaters Anonymous. Such a group can serve three valuable functions. First, it may offer ideas about sound weight loss tactics, low calorie foods, and recipes. Second, it can offer a discipline, a structured approach to follow. Third, it may provide positive reinforcement in the form of praise for success and encouragement when we are low. Good ideas, discipline, and reinforcement are valuable aids to a dieter.

Additionally, you may find the routine of attending a diet club or peer support group periodically, and sharing experiences with others dealing with the same problems you are, helpful as another reminder keeping your energy focused on weight control. The helpfulness to you of the organization will depend upon your compatibility with the group's philosophy and methods, the particular leader or specialist with whom you are in contact, and the other people with whom you are sharing the experience. If it works for you, do it. But remember, only you can do the job. You are the miracle. Eventually, you will almost assuredly stop going to the club or group. Then more than ever be sure this book is close by. If you will just absorb what is being said in this book, you won't need any other teacher.

It is imperative to see that weight control is not a diet. In fact, thinking of it as a diet is counterproductive. A diet conjures up the image of something unpleasant, regimented, even painful. We are engaging in something else—something that is fun, stimulating, and challenging. Something that will last. A game that makes us feel good. And a game that, if you will play it, will change the course of your life for the better. We are involved in taking charge of our bodies and finding out that we really can control them. This opens up enormous opportunities for affecting our health, our moods, and our mastery of the environment in which we live.

[27]

The Mathematics of Weight Control

IN ORDER TO UNDERSTAND what gaining and losing weight is all about, one needs to think in terms of calories. Technically speaking, a calorie is the amount of heat needed to raise the temperature of one kilogram of water one degree Centigrade. But for our purposes, we need only think of calories as a measurement of the energy-producing value of food. The energy that is in the food we eat is either used by the body for its current activity or, if not so used, the energy is converted to and stored by the body as fat. Food is converted into energy that the body either uses now or stores for possible future use. When the amount of energy (calories) in the food a person eats is greater than the amount of calories of energy his or her body is currently expending, the person puts on weight. Conversely, if the body uses more calories of energy than it is getting from the food eaten, the body draws upon some of the energy stored as fat to make up for the shortfall, and the person loses weight.

The only way to lose weight is to eat less calories than one is expending as energy in one's daily routine.

It is generally accepted that a pound consists of approximately 3,500 calories. This means that if over some period of time one eats 3,500 calories more in food than he or she expends in energy, at the end of the period, the person will weigh one whole pound more than at the beginning of the period. On the other hand, if during some period of time, one expends 3,500 calories of energy more than he or she receives from the food eaten, at the end of the period, the person will weigh one full pound less. Either using more calories of energy or eating less calories of food will result in losing weight.

Theoretically armed with the above knowledge, it should be simple to calculate *how long* it will take to lose one pound. First, one would ascertain *how many calories of food* are needed each day to keep his or her weight *exactly* at its current level. Second, he or she would decide how many calories *less* than that number to eat each day. Third, by dividing the number of calories deducted each day into 3,500, one would calculate *how many days* it would take to lose one pound. For example, let us say that a person who wants to lose ten pounds ascertains that when he or she eats 2,500 calories a day, his or her weight remains perfectly level. If the person decides to eat 500 calories less a day (2,000 instead of 2,500), this person should lose one pound every seven days (500 calories a day divided into 3,500 calories equals seven days). And it should take (10 x 7) 70 days or ten weeks to reach the 10-pound weight loss goal.

Unfortunately, as is often the case in life, theory is difficult to apply in the real world. The first problem is that it is not easy to ascertain exactly how many calories of energy one is using each day. There is no precise guide to rely on. It depends on a number of factors, including age, sex, lifestyle, metabolism, physical activity, and current weight. And the number of calories will change as a person's weight changes. We only really can find out how many calories of energy we use each day if we laboriously tinker with our calorie intake, fine tuning it to a point where our weight doesn't fluctuate; count the calories we are eating over a period of four or five days; and then compute a daily average. It isn't worth the effort.

The second problem in applying the mathematical theory of weight loss to the realities of life is that it is very difficult to calculate with real accuracy the number of calories we consume in a day unless we scrupulously measure the quantity of every food we eat. And even then, there are problems. I do not measure the foods that I eat in order to count calories. I simply make estimates based on experience. Notwithstanding what may seem like a casual approach to counting calories, I cannot emphasize enough how important it is to count your calories every day. Remembering the right things at the right moment; making your list; always eating when you are hungry; and counting calories are the cornerstones of a successful weight control program. I have a lot of experience estimating quantities and I know the approximate number of calories in the foods I eat. If at first it will help, measure what you eat with a food scale and measuring cup and keep a written record of the results. You won't do it forever, but a few weeks of measuring and writing down the food and the amount of calories in it will soon make you a skillful estimator of the number of calories you are eating. (The calories contained in almost all foods can be found in the listing at the back of this book.)

At the outset of your program, you need to set a daily calorie target that is consistent either with your losing weight or maintaining your weight at its current level. In setting this target, you will at first also have to do some estimating. As a rough rule of thumb, it takes approximately 15 calories in food a day to supply the energy needed to maintain each pound we weigh. This means that if a person weighs 200 pounds, and if the rule were precisely accurate, if the person ate 200 x 15 or 3,000 calories each day, his or her weight would remain at exactly 200 pounds. Eating less than an average of 3,000 calories a day would result in losing weight, while eating more than an average of 3,000 calories each day would result in gaining weight. To apply the rule of thumb to yourself, you need only multiply your current weight times fifteen. You will then know, very approximately, how many calories you can eat on the average each day to maintain your weight at its current level. The chart on the next page is constructed according to this rule of thumb and will save your having to do the multiplication.

Average Number of Calories Per Day
Needed to Maintain a Person's Weight

Pounds	Calories	Pounds	Calories	Pounds	Calories
100	1500	135	2025	170	2550
105	1575	140	2100	175	2625
110	1650	145	2175	180	2700
115	1725	150	2250	185	2775
120	1800	155	2325	190	2850
125	1875	160	2400	195	2925
130	1950	165	2475	200	3000

I want to stress again that the numbers in the above chart are only approximations and that any person's individual experience may vary quite significantly from this general guide. For example, age will make a difference—possibly a big difference. According to another rough rule of thumb, after age twenty-five, a person's calorie needs drop nearly one percent a year. Thus at age fifty, the number of calories needed to maintain a person's weight might be 20 percent less than the number needed at age twenty-five. But so much depends on individual characteristics and lifestyle that nothing can be taken for granted. However, we can use the chart or the rule of thumb it is based on in setting an initial calorie target; a place to start.

I suggest that in the weight loss phase, you set your initial calorie target as 25 to 50 percent fewer calories than the number the chart indicates is needed to keep your weight stable at the level that you have set as your goal. Not at your *present* weight, but rather at your *goal* weight. Thus, if you weighed 150 pounds and you wanted to weigh 130 pounds, you would subtract the 25 to 50 percent from the 1,950 calories required to keep your weight at your goal of 130 pounds, not from the 2,250 calories necessary to keep your weight at its current 150-pound level. (Your daily target would be somewhere between 975 and 1,465 calories.) However, never set a target of less than 1,000 calories a day without first discussing it with your doctor.

When you begin your weight control program, if you feel it necessary, you can weigh yourself once a week for the first two weeks—just to be sure you are losing weight. But beware of being carried away by the substantial weight loss registered in this first week or two. Much of this early weight loss is an illusion. Most of these initially lost pounds are just water draining from the body, not burned off fat. The first week's weight loss should be between two and ten pounds, depending on personal characteristics and how overweight you are. The second week's loss will be less substantial. By the third week, the results will probably be pretty paltry and you should be nearing what your average weight loss will be in the period ahead. All is well as long as you are losing weight at the end of week two. Your calorie target is reasonable and you are staying within it. Stop using the scale for the reasons I have outlined in the chapter "Hide the Scale."

If you want to lose more weight than you are now losing, you must either lower your daily calorie target or increase your energy expenditure, or do both. If you have not been losing any weight, either you are not counting your daily calorie intake reasonably accurately, or your daily calorie target is too high. First, check your calorie counting. Every day for a week, write down each thing you eat and its calorie value. Add the daily calorie count accurately. If this detailed analysis proves that you have been accurately counting your daily calorie intake; then and only then; lower your daily calorie target. I will talk more about dealing with this contingency in Chapter 29, "If It Isn't Working."

In order to fully understand the mathematics of weight control, one need consider three periods of time: the very beginning, the middle, and the end of the weight loss phase of the program. As I indicated, due to the illusory effect of the body's loss of water, the beginning of the weight loss period is a heady time. There is a relatively quick weight loss. This rapid loss in weeks one and two will happen naturally whenever one takes action to lose weight, no matter what that action may be. It is this natural bodily phenomenon that all the fad diets capitalize on in their advertisements about how quickly they will make you lose five to ten pounds. But these liquid pounds are always lurking about ready to pile back on in as big a hurry as they were lost. The major part of this early big weight loss has not come from using up energy stored as fat.

The middle phase of the weight loss period is one of slow, methodical burning up of the body's fat. As the weight loss increases, our body's need for energy gradually decreases. There is that much less weight to lug around, cause to move, and take care of. *Each pound lost decreases by about 15 calories the amount of energy the body needs to do its day's work.* Thus, after having lost five, ten, twenty, thirty pounds, if you are still eating the same number of calories per day as when you first started your program, your weight loss will be progressively slower. For example, after losing twenty pounds, it will take 300 (20 x 15) fewer calories per day to match your energy expenditure. That's 2,100 calories (or close to two-thirds of a pound) a week less weight loss than when you started. This decline in the number of calories needed to keep one's weight level as the diet progresses is a major reason why weight loss gets slower as the dieter moves closer to his or her goal, closer to the end of the weight loss phase of the program.

A second reason is that as we lose weight due to eating less, there is a tendency for the body to lower its thermostat and to begin to require even less fuel. This tendency will be seen vividly in people who go on starvation diets for long periods of time. Their weight loss will be much less than expected because their body has adjusted its energy needs drastically downward. A third reason is that as we keep going, buoyed by success, if we are not vigilant, we may tend to eat a little more here, a little more there, and our calorie intake increases ever so slightly, thus compounding the slowdown.

It is important for our psychological well-being that we truly understand the nasty tricks the retention of water can play on our weight. Weight loss occurs in a stepwise pattern like a staircase rather than in a level, consistent downgrade like a ramp. Our body seems to pause at new levels of lower body weight before taking the next step down. During these pauses, on a day to-day basis, the scale may even show us gaining a pound or so. As long as you have not been inadvertently eating more calories than you have targeted for, this gain is almost certainly due to the retention of water by fat tissue. During weight loss periods, water often accumulates, particularly in middle-aged and older women. This occurs because the skin and subsurface tissue have not shrunk as fast as the fat has been lost. The empty spaces become filled with water, which will be lost as the skin and underlying tissue shrink.

This water-retention phenomenon will affect different people in extremely different ways. A person may lose two pounds one day, not lose weight for five days, gain a pound or two, and then two days later, lose five pounds as the accumulated water is lost. Another person may not lose any weight for ten days and then in the next day or two, lose seven pounds. It is because this erratic and totally unpredictable fluctuating in one's weight can at times be so depressing that I think periodic weighings are very dangerous.

Understanding the mathematics of weight control is very useful because it provides a simple, workable framework in which to think about gaining, losing, or maintaining weight. Using a daily calorie target offers both a guide in selecting what to eat, as well as a way of exercising self-discipline. And taking time to count calories serves as another reminder, helping to keep weight control in the forefront of consciousness. Thus I faithfully count calories every day. But I don't let my calorie target obsess me. I establish a daily calorie guide, but I rarely hit it. I concentrate on the type of foods I am eating. I use the guide to check that I am not continuously exceeding my targeted calorie intake. I know the approximate calorie value of the foods I eat, and I concentrate heavily on the low calorie foods that I like. I pay attention to calories and I set guidelines, but my focus is on the type of food that I am eating, not on an absolutely accurate calorie count of everything that I put in my stomach. This approach can be dangerous if you don't truly stick to low calorie foods or if you deceive yourself. What I am saying is use the calorie target, but don't let it obsess you.

I think the idea of setting a fixed, inviolate number of calories that one must meet each day is self-defeating. If I eat more than my allotted calories, I will feel badly, as if I have failed. And conversely, the attitude of many dieters that if they have eaten less than their allotted number, they can reward themselves with something high in calories, can be even more damaging. There is no need to punish yourself or feel guilty if on some days you exceed a reasonable standard by a couple of hundred calories as long as you have been following the basic commandments of eating when you are hungry and only eating nonfattening foods you like the taste of.

Nor is there any reason to reward yourself if you have eaten less calories than you have targeted for. I think the technique of banking calories now to give yourself a treat later is as counterproductive as is punishing yourself for eating too many calories. Banking calories goes like this: If you are allowing yourself 1,500 calories per day and you have only eaten 1,000, then you have 500 calories left at night to use in any way that you like. Or possibly, you eat 200 calories a day less than your daily allotment so that at the end of a week you have 1,400 calories in the bank for a rich treat. Banking calories sums up a self-defeating frame of mind. This technique encourages people engaged in weight control to see themselves as deprived, which, when weight control is pursued properly, they are not. If you eat when you are hungry and the things you eat taste good, you are not deprived. Your hunger urge is being satisfied just as effectively, possibly more effectively, than if you were eating one of those fattening goodies that people are binging on with the calories they have banked. If you are hungry, eat. If you are not, don't. If you eat fewer calories in a day than your guide calls for, that's fine, so long as you have eaten when you are hungry. These lesser-calorie days make up for those other days that you go over the limit. You are that much further ahead of the game. To treat yourself to a rich dessert or some other fattening goodie as a reward is only going to tempt you to stray from the path. Remember, tastes feed on themselves. The second bite is harder to avoid than is the first. It isn't useful to give yourself a treat by eating things that you are trying to diminish your taste for. The longer you stay away from, and the less you eat of, those rich foods that still tempt you, the less they will tempt you later on. The less important they will seem. If you want to give yourself a treat for being so good that will make you feel terrific in a constructive way, buy something to wear that will make your new, slimmer figure look even more attractive to you. Or if you prefer, pamper your body with a massage, or a bubble bath. These sources of feeling good will reinforce your weight control program, not undermine it the way that eating fattening treats as a reward is almost certain to do.

[28]

What to Do

THIS CHAPTER DETAILS THE PLAN that will make effortless, enjoyable, weight control a reality for you. This chapter tells you what to do to make effective weight control just happen naturally. It summarizes and organizes those things discussed in the preceding chapters that will empower you to successfully control your weight. When you look at this plan, you will see just how simple weight control is going to be. How very little there is to do. But you have to do it, or it won't work. Do each and every one of the following things. Don't skip any.

1. If you have not yet done so, set your goal; the number of pounds you would like to lose and the weight you would like to maintain. (Chapter 3)

2. Write out the reason (or reasons) you want to control your weight. Take some time doing this. Try to get in touch with your reason by feeling the desire it arouses in you. (Chapter 6)

3. Buy a small looseleaf notebook. Carry it with you at all times in a pocket or purse. The purpose of this notebook is to assist you in remembering essential things that will give birth to and then nurture your weight control program. (The reason that this notebook should be looseleaf is for convenience, so that you can insert new pages in appropriate sections.)

4. In this notebook, list those low calorie foods, beverages, and food combinations that you find tasty, or at least acceptable. (For convenience, list snacks separate from meals.) From this list, you can select at any time a Low Calorie Solution to the challenge posed by an urge to eat. Making this list and adding new ideas to it is a most crucial part of creating and maintaining your weight control program. Put a copy of this list on both your refrigerator and your food cupboard doors, and keep these copies updated as you add new ideas. (Chapters 6 and 7)

5. In a separate section of this notebook, write down anything you notice about your reactions to food. Examples of items that I have noted in this section are: "I lost my appetite while I was watching the movie about open-heart surgery"; "When I exercise hard, my appetite diminishes, but when I exercise lightly, my appetite increases"; "I really felt uncomfortable after eating all that apple pie at Thanksgiving dinner"; "When I drank coffee with sugar in it, it satisfied my urge to eat a chocolate ice cream sundae. I felt perfectly comfortable and glad I hadn't eaten the sundae." Once a week reread any notes you have made in this section. This weekly review will keep you in touch with those fragments of insight you have about your relation to food and will help you in creating and maintaining your weight control program. (Chapter 9)

6. In a third section of this notebook, each day list the approximate number of calories you have eaten that day. This calorie counting exercise serves a number of purposes besides allowing you to judge whether you are eating approximately the number of calories you want to be eating. It will get you into and keep you in the habit of counting calories, which is a vital part of the "Keeping It Off" phase of your weight control program. It will give you a record to refer to if you need to make any adjustments in your weight control program. And, finally, it will serve as another reminder of weight control that will help bring to consciousness those essential ideas discussed in Chapter 5 that need to be remembered each time we begin to eat. (Chapter 27) When making this daily entry as to the number of calories eaten, take a few moments to review the day and see if you want to record anything in the section of the notebook relating to your reactions to food.

7. Set a daily calorie limit for yourself. In initially setting this limit, refer to the chart on page 133, and deduct 25 to 50 percent from the number of calories indicated as necessary to maintain your goal weight (not your current weight). (Chapter 27)

8. Write on six large index cards in bold, capital letters, in clear, dark print:

A. You want to control your weight because (fill in your reason).

B. You will feel worse if you overeat than if you don't.

C. You will choose the Low Calorie Solution.

Put one of these cards on the door of your refrigerator, another on the door of your food cupboard, a third in the middle of the bathroom mirror, and the others in places at work, at home, or in your car, where you will see them frequently. (Chapter 6)

9. Reread parts of this book for ten minutes each day. Keep this book with you until you are really secure that you are effectively in charge of your weight control program. Reading this book daily will help you remember the right thing at the right time, stimulate new, positive ideas in your mind, and keep your energy aroused and channeled to weight control. It is repeated exposure to the right message that will make your program a success. The mind will go where it is directed to go. And we will go where our mind goes. If you are having trouble getting started, concentrate on Chapters 8 and 13, "Starting" and "Intention Makes It Happen." Once you have begun, concentrate on Chapters 17

and 13, "Midstream" and "Intention Makes it Happen." If you have reached your goal, concentrate on Chapters 22 and 13, "Keeping it Off" and "Intention Makes it Happen." Of course, you should also read from other sections of this book. Those chapters I have singled out are of particular significance at the different points indicated along the path to weight control. Just having this book with you and seeing it will help jolt you into remembering the right thing at the right moment. (Chapter 6)

10. Say to yourself slowly each morning when you awaken and each night before bed, "I would really feel and look good if I lost _____ pounds and kept my weight at _____." (You fill in the blanks in accord with the goal you have selected in number 1 above.) Tape a reminder to do this over the face of the clock nearest your bed so that anytime you want to see this clock, which most of us do first thing in the morning and before going to sleep, you will have to see this reminder and lift it so as to read the time. (Chapter 3)

11. Before each meal, slowly say to yourself, twice, "During this meal, I will remember that I want to control my weight because_____." (You fill in the blank in accord with the reason or reasons you wrote in response to number 2 above.) "I will feel badly if I overeat and I do not want to continue eating after my stomach is full." "I want to choose the Low Calorie Solution." Before each snack, ask yourself slowly, "Am I really hungry? Is this the Low Calorie Solution?" It is essential to say these things slowly and allow yourself to dwell on them for a few moments. Keep saying these things even if you are not yet choosing the Low Calorie Solution. Realize that the words are designed to focus your consciousness; to make you stop and think; to have you focusing on weight control when you begin eating. The words won't do it for you. But the words will lead you to do it, naturally, effortlessly. It takes some people longer than others. Just keep raising your weight control consciousness at meals and snacktimes, and do the other things I am suggesting. After a while, it will work. It will happen naturally. Just keep on jogging your memory. (Chapter 6)

12. Once a day, read or recite from memory the following:

A. Use the Law of Deflection. (Chapter 11)

B. Use the Law of Distraction. (Chapter 10)

C. Think about what you will eat when you are planning not to be eating at home and if necessary, take an acceptable low calorie food with you. (Chapter 21)

D. Never shop for food while you are hungry. To the greatest extent possible, buy only low calorie foods and don't buy foods to which you are addicted. Look for new low calorie ideas to add to your list. (Chapter 24)

E. Exercise, while not necessary, will be a big plus in a weight control program. (Chapter 25)

After you have reached your goal, do the following: (Chapter 22)

1. Continue to count calories each day; say those things we have been saying before meals and snacks; keep your list up to date.

2. Change what you say every morning when you awaken and every evening before bed to: "I will keep my weight at _____ pounds."

3. Weigh yourself at least once a week.

4. If you are ever more than three pounds over your goal, immediately return to the weight loss phase of the program. Immediately! Not tomorrow or Monday!

5. After you have maintained your goal for a month, you can take down the index card on the bathroom mirror. Leave the others in place. You can also stop reading this book, but put it somewhere that you can see it frequently, such as on a living room coffee table or on the nightstand near your bed.

6. After two months of maintaining your goal, you can stop reading the list in number 12 above, and you need only refer to the notes about your reactions to food once every two months or so.

That's all you need to do to implement a successful weight control program. Buy a notebook. Create a list. Write a few sentences on six index cards. Set a daily calorie guide and count calories on a daily basis. Say a few words in the morning, at night, and before meals and snacks. Read this book, and refer to a brief list of reminders. Then it will happen naturally. Just let it!

Remember, any tendency to shortcut, to believe "I don't have to do each and every one of these things and keep doing them" is the beginning of your creating roadblocks to your success. It is the *doing* of the concrete acts as I am outlining them that will keep *stimulating* the proper mindset. Not just at first when you may be full of enthusiasm, but later on as the initial enthusiasm wanes. Often in all areas of life, the difference between success and failure is nothing more than paying attention to details. Do each and every thing I am suggesting unless you have a better idea as how to really control your weight.

[29]

If It Isn't Working

WHAT DO YOU DO if you think you have really, truly (cross your heart) done everything I have suggested in this book, and you have not started to lose weight? This problem can come in two forms. Either a person is trying, but not losing weight, or a person has not yet even begun to try. Either a person has reduced his or her calorie intake below the number of calories he or she believes they are expending each day, and there has been no weight loss; or the person experiencing the problem has not yet even felt moved to begin to control his or her weight, as I say he or she must, simply by doing what I suggest.

Let's start with the person who is already trying, but not losing weight. Unless you have some metabolic or other physical uniqueness, and probably even then, if you are not losing weight, or even worse, you are gaining it, it is for one reason and one reason alone. You are taking in more calories than your body is burning. I once read a story in a popular news magazine about a very fat person in a circus who went on a diet. Before going on the diet, this person used to eat an unbelievably enormous amount of food each day—something like six loaves of bread, six chickens, six milkshakes, etc. On the diet, the person ate about half of what he normally consumed: three loaves of bread, three chickens, three milkshakes. After a week, the person weighed himself and found that he had gained two pounds. Discouraged, he gave up the diet. True, this person had cut his food intake substantially, but the food he was eating still had more calories than his body was using. So he gained weight even though he had reduced his food intake.

If you think you are cutting down on your calorie intake sufficiently to lose weight, and you are not losing weight, the first thing to do, as the scientists would say, is to "Check your assumptions." You need to find out if you really have cut your calorie intake as much as you are estimating. In order to do this, you need to become more serious about counting calories than heretofore. The rough approximations that are usually adequate will not do. You must increase the accuracy of your count. To accomplish this, you need to know the exact size of the portions that you eat and the calorie count for that size portion. In order to measure portions accurately, you will need to obtain a food scale and a measuring cup. The calorie count for most foods can be found at the end of this book.

First, weigh yourself. Then continue eating as you have been doing. Continue to eat the number of calories you believe you have been eating, the amount you have assigned as your daily target. Don't change anything. But now write down each thing that you eat, the quantity, and the number of calories it contains. At this point, you are not just interested in calculating the daily total. You also want to record as much detail as possible so you can analyze what you are eating in order to see what adjustments can be made. An illustration of such detailed calorie counting for two days will be found in Appendix B.

After a week, weigh yourself again. Not any sooner! Daily fluctuations can be very misleading. Are you losing weight now? If so, you apparently had been eating more calories than you thought you had. Once you started tracking your calories carefully, you automatically reduced your intake to the target level. You need only keep doing what you have done over the last week. For a while, at least, keep recording the calories in each thing you eat in scrupulous detail. This recording procedure has proven to be an important assist in keeping your calorie counting accurate. And the detailed record may be of value in analyzing where you are going astray, if in a future period you are not losing weight as you reasonably expect you should be. The record will enable you to compare what you were eating when you were losing weight with what you are eating later, when you are not.

But if you are not losing weight at the end of this one-week period, you now know that you must either cut your calorie intake target or increase your energy output. Possibly a little of both. Cutting calories will mean that you must concentrate more than you have been on those foods, beverages, and food combinations that are at the lower calorie end of your list of acceptably tasty, nonfattening foods.

Analyze the list of foods that you have been eating. How could you make adjustments that would increase your consumption of the lower calorie foods and decrease your intake of the higher calorie ones? Think about substituting lower calorie items for more fattening choices. Appendix B gives examples of substitutes for some foods that will lower the number of calories consumed with little or no sacrifice in real satisfaction. Once when I was trying to cut some calories from my already reduced level, I took the eggs off a lunchtime salad I was often having at a salad bar, decreased the amount of Jell-O on it, and added some broccoli. What might you substitute for the higher-calorie foods? Think about it. It is simply a problem to be unraveled—a problem that you can easily solve with imagination and intention.

One way to think about the problem is to find combining tastes that make lower calorie foods acceptably tasty. While the chart in Appendix A lumps a lot of foods together and classifies them as nonfattening, in reality some of these foods have considerably more calories than do others. For instance, let's compare celery and sweet cherries. An ounce of celery has a lot fewer calories than does an ounce of sweet cherries. Your stomach will be filled considerably more by a quantity of celery containing 50 calories than by cherries containing the same number of calories. Find combining tastes that make the lower calorie foods acceptable. For example, I put a little ricotta or cottage cheese, some diet jam, or possibly a little salt on celery (though I do try not to eat much salt these days).

Remember, there is another way to approach the problem; namely, by increasing the number of calories you use. For example, walking briskly for half an hour a day, preferably but not necessarily before dinner, will help both in using calories and reducing appetite. But the walking or any other exercise you do must be relatively strenuous for your physical state. While heavy exercise diminishes hunger, light exercise may well increase your appetite. (But remember, no strenuous exercise before you talk to your doctor about what you intend to do.)

For some people, losing weight seems to be more difficult than for others. But for everyone, it can really be easy, if you will tune into what I am saying and faithfully do what I am suggesting. You simply need to discover and cultivate your taste for low calorie foods, beverages, and food combinations, and to avoid the addictive foods that are causing you to gain weight. Even if you must cut down another few hundred calories a day, good tastes are still available, and you need never be hungry. So there is no reason to feel discouraged and quit.

Now let's deal with the second form of the "It's not working" problem—the person who has not yet even felt moved to begin trying. You need to do three things. First, truly answer the question, have you really done everything I have suggested? Everything? Are you saying those things you are supposed to before each meal, each snack, before bed and in the morning? Are you making your list of satisfying low calorie foods? Have you posted it on your refrigerator and food cupboard doors? Are you reading from this book each day, and reading or reciting daily the list in number 12 in Chapter 28? Have you made and posted your index cards? Are you counting calories every day? If you have been doing these things, keep doing them and also add these two exercises.

1. After each meal or snack, ask yourself, "How could I have done it differently, in a nonfattening but still satisfying manner?" In order to remind yourself to ask this question, write it on a piece of paper and tape it to your dining room table. Write out your answers to the question. Write out those low calorie foods you could have eaten that would have been enjoyable and the number of calories in these foods. Also write out the number of calories in the meal or snack you have just had. By constantly critiquing your actions in this way, you will begin to see new possibilities that will make it work for you.

2. After each meal or snack, imagine what you would tell someone else who said to you they wanted to lose weight and asked you for advice as to what they should do. Tell it to them, tell it to them good. Out loud! By teaching this imaginary person, you will be programming yourself.

If you really intend to control your weight, then by doing the things I suggest, you will get your mind into the right gear. It may take time, possibly quite some time. But when your mind is set, the details will fall into place. That's right—the details will fall into place. You will do what is necessary to reach and maintain the goal you have set for yourself. But remember, it all starts with intention. And you prove your intention by scrupulously doing each thing that I have suggested and by not giving up.

[30]

Basic Principles

IN CHAPTER 3, I said that in this book I was going to explain both the basic principles of painless, effective, enjoyable weight control and the tactics I have used to successfully implement these principles. The principles are etched in stone and inviolate. My tactics are personal and can be varied, simplified, supplemented, or disregarded to suit your personal tastes. The following are the basic principles:

1. Always eat when you are hungry.

2. Tailor-make your own weight control program to your own likes and dislikes. Don't go on someone else's diet.

3. Begin by selecting a weight goal for yourself.
   A. Create reminders that will bring this goal to your mind repeatedly.

   B. Reach your goal—don't let up after a good start.

4. Get in touch with why you want to lose weight; how badly you will feel if you eat imprudently; the low calorie foods you like.
   A. Bring the idea of weight control to your mind frequently and especially when you are about to begin eating by creating reminders to yourself of why you

want to lose weight; how badly you will feel if you eat imprudently; and that there is always a Low Calorie Solution to your hunger.

5. Deflect the urge for fattening foods.

6. Create and maintain your intention by surrounding yourself with weight control and thereby coming to understand in your bones that it is very important and easy.

7. Don't be in a hurry to lose weight.

8. Keep fattening foods to which you are addicted out of the house, or if this is not possible, then under lock and key (with someone else in possession of the key).

9. Set a daily calorie target and count the calories you eat each day.

10. Don't let unusual situations such as parties, eating out, or vacations serve as an excuse for eating imprudently. If possible, plan ahead; if not possible, use your creativity, and be flexible.

11. Keep the weight off by continuing to count calories, using reminders and adding to your list of low calorie foods and food combinations you enjoy.

[31]

Keep Your Eye on the Ball

I HAVE STRESSED throughout this book that what I have come to understand is simple for you to learn. Our minds control our actions. And our minds work on the principle of associating ideas. All that needs to be done to turn fat into slim is, when we are confronted with hunger, to set the association chain in the mind going in a different and positive direction, the direction we really want to go in. We do this by using the hunger urge to remind us to say those things we have learned to say before eating: (1) why we want to lose weight; (2) that if we overeat we will feel worse than if we do not; and (3) there is a Low Calorie Solution to our momentary hunger urge that will alleviate the bodily sensation we are feeling just as effectively as a more fattening one. In this way, and by exposing ourselves frequently to other brief reminders, we program our minds to direct us to effortless weight control. The repeated memories will have their effect. You will automatically first lose weight and then keep your weight under control—maybe not immediately, but certainly in time.

Don't quit! That is the important thing. The longer you keep doing something, the more real it becomes. What I have told you will work whether you want to lose 5 or 105 pounds. Better still, it will keep the pounds off and rid you of your addictions to food. Just do the things I have suggested in order to stimulate your memory. It is really that easy. I know it is hard for you to believe. It may seem ridiculous that making a list, saying a few words repeatedly, rereading this book, and a couple of other simple, undramatic acts are going to make you accomplish what you have failed at so often before. But while these acts may seem like nothing, they are in fact everything. Everything necessary to make weight control a reality. I have tried to demonstrate that I have gone through what you are going through by telling you of my experiences, even if some of them did not show me off as I might like to be seen. I have done this so you will say to yourself, "Maybe he really knows what he is talking about, even if I don't see it yet."

If it doesn't work at first for you, get up each time you fall. Be gentle with yourself. Don't struggle! But keep going! Think about how you might be doing it differently in order to make it work. Today may be the day it works. The day your engine turns over.

I have also stressed that you need never be hungry and you can have lots of good tastes; that there are many low calorie foods and food combinations with satisfying tastes that will alleviate your urge to eat fattening foods just as effectively as if you had eaten a fattening food. I have not told you that you can eat hot fudge sundaes or other tempting delights that pile on the pounds. You can't! That's the bad news! The good news is that you can create your own nonfattening food satisfactions if you allow your creativity to take charge and don't stubbornly insist they taste exactly like the fattening delights. They may not. But the important thing is that they will do the job as effectively. And in time you will prefer their taste to the taste of the addictive foods you are now eating. It may take some experimentation to get in touch with those nonfattening tastes you enjoy. But the satisfying tastes are there. Remember, all tastes have been acquired, though some more readily than others.

Weight control is a skill just like driving a car is a skill. Just like driving a car, this skill takes some time to learn and requires some practice. Unfortunately, unlike when you learn to drive a car, there is no one sitting right next to you to guide you step by step through the learning process, making suggestions and correcting your mistakes. I think this book and my cassette tapes are the closest thing you are going to find to a person sitting beside you who really understands what you are going through, and can tell you how to meet the problems you are encountering. That is why I tell you to keep the book close and reread it until you have absorbed its message, until its message is internalized into your body. Until you have internalized the message, keep me with you to help deal with those moments when the enthusiasm you felt may be temporarily dampened.

Eventually, you will be your own teacher, and in fact, you know the entire teaching. All you need do is to effectively organize what you know so you can communicate it to yourself in a manner that is intelligible. That is what made weight control a reality for me. I learned how to organize and communicate to myself, in a truly understandable manner, things that I already knew. You can do the same thing. It may help if you picture yourself telling someone else what to do. What would you tell someone else to do at this particular moment, if his or her body were behaving as yours is now behaving? Possibly you would tell him or her that all one need learn is which low calorie foods he or she likes in order to make the discomfort of hunger vanish in a constructive rather than a destructive manner. Possibly you would say, go out and try the Law of Deflection and the Law of Distraction for yourself. See how these principles really work. Possibly you would say, you can addict yourself to weight control simply by surrounding yourself with it.

Another thing I have stressed is that the best way to get the acknowledgement that will reinforce your energy and enthusiasm is to focus on how you are feeling and how your clothes are fitting. It is the constant feel of yourself, the lightness, the greater aliveness pulsating within, that will overwhelm those forces trying to make you backtrack into the heaviness and sluggishness that tends to deaden overweight people. It's nice to hear other people praise your weight loss, but the words quickly vanish, while the good bodily feeling is always there.

A fourth part of the message is that there is no hurry. It is much better to lose weight slowly. At times it might seem like nothing much is happening, but every moment helps to weaken the hypnotic spell that conditions our behavior around food. If you become discouraged, don't let up! Think about how you can change what you are doing.

If you have read this far and you are not hepped up enough to begin, ask yourself, "Why don't I act?" Probably because you think it is hard and unpleasant, or because you think you can't. Neither is true. It is not hard and unpleasant and you certainly can. Why can't you? Life is going to be better if you control your weight. Just follow my suggestions and let your creativity take charge. The ideas will flow into your head. The journey of a thousand miles begins with one step. But beware of starting with a big burst of enthusiasm, then petering out and putting this book away. If you start to falter, get back in touch with your intention. Revive your intention. Keep in touch with your intention. Feel your desire! Raise your energy!

I have said that weight control is a creative act. Certainly this is so. First, it is creative in the sense that one designs the process for oneself by finding those low calorie foods he or she likes and by making these foods taste good. But in a larger sense we can create the way our lives are going to be. *What I am today is a result of what I did yesterday. What you are tomorrow is a result of what you do today.* It is an act of creativity to make something happen that wouldn't otherwise have happened except for the fact that you did something. You create a weight control program that will last for the rest of your life simply by beginning. You start somewhere, some time, simply by creating a beginning. By taking the first step. There are no trumpets blaring, lights flashing, or bells ringing when you take the first steps to change the course of your life. But you can do that on any day, at any moment. And this moment is as good as any other you will ever find for creating the beginning of your weight control program.

We are at the end of this book, but I hope not at the end of our relationship. That, I hope, is just beginning. People need friends to help and support them. The best friends, of course, are real life ones, in the flesh; those whom we know personally. But I am a real person, in the flesh, and I understand. A book is really one person talking to another, telling a story or explaining something. Stay in touch with me as you would a friend. Keep me with you by rereading this book a number of times. If you don't reread it, you will forget this book, as I have forgotten so many books which I read in order to learn to do things I still want to learn to do. In rereading these pages you will absorb, internalize my message. Then you will always hear my voice reminding you, as it reminds me, that there is a Low Calorie Solution to the momentary hunger we are feeling. In that way we will go on together forever.

Afterword

ALTHOUGH FROM THE STANDPOINT of feeling good, looking good, staying healthy, and living longer, proper nutrition is a handmaiden of weight control, this book does not deal directly with nutritional issues. Good nutrition does overlap and may even correspond identically with weight control in promoting a good looking, good feeling, healthy body. But notwithstanding this close relationship, this possible identity, nutrition and weight control are in fact separate skills.

First, let me say that it is possible to do everything that I suggest in this book in a way that is totally consistent with ideal nutrition. You will just tailor-make your diet accordingly. Secondly, it really is impossible to continually implement a Low Calorie Solution that allows you to eat whenever you are hungry if you do not eat in a fairly sound manner. You will just naturally eat fruits, vegetables, and cereals, and abstain from high fat, high sugar, and junk foods. While this won't always guarantee the ideal nutritional balance, it will keep you pointed in the right direction.

My belief is that if one has had difficulty in truly controlling his or her weight, he or she can come to weight control with proper nutrition much more quickly and much more assuredly by first learning the skill of weight control, rather than vice versa, or trying to learn both skills at once.

If you learn the skill of weight control, the skill of good nutrition will rather easily follow. And beware of using a proper desire for good nutrition to serve as an improper excuse for not acting effectively to control your weight. You can eat nutritiously and be fat. The real benefit of good nutrition is diluted considerably if you are overweight.

In mastering the skill of weight control as I am teaching it, one learns things that can be used in meeting other problems of life and learning other skills, including good nutrition. For example, in beginning to notice one's bodily urges and one's bodily energies, you will begin to notice the effect that different foods are having on your energy and your moods.

If we try to do too much at once, biting off more than we can chew, so to speak, we often become overwhelmed. For most people, a toe at a time is a better approach than trying to do it all at once. We usually need to focus attention one step at a time. Body and mind adapt slowly. Most people can't start from scratch and begin running five miles a day. Most of us would have to build to it gradually or we would unwisely and unproductively overstress our bodies. There is a great danger that our attention will become distracted, that we will be overwhelmed, possibly confused, and we will feel overstressed if we try to learn the skills of weight control and nutrition both at once.

After you have gotten your weight under control, the awareness that you are gaining in tailor-making your own diet, and the desire to keep feeling good, possibly even better, will most probably lead you naturally along the path of wanting to also master the skill of nutrition. That has been my experience. In time I think everyone should gradually incorporate the skill of nutrition into their weight control program. Some ways of controlling one's weight are a lot smarter than are others.

Appendix A

LOW CALORIE FOODS

The following can be eaten in very large quantities without disrupting a weight control program. Where necessary, taste satisfaction can be easily enhanced in a nonfattening manner. Use this list to begin compiling your own list of personally satisfying low calorie foods.

	Cal. Per Oz.		Cal. Per Oz.
Apples	16	Green Beans	9
Apricots	14	Honeydew (diced)	10
Artichokes	3	Honeydew (melon)	6
Asparagus	6	Mustard Greens	7
Bean Sprouts	10	Okra	9
Beets	9	Onions	11
Beet Greens	5	Oranges	10
Blackberries	13	Papaya (diced)	11
Blueberries	18	Papaya (whole)	7
Boysenberries	10	Peaches	10
Broccoli	8	Pears	17
Brussel Sprouts	10	Peppers (sweet)	5
Cabbage	6	Pickles (dill/sour)	3
Cantaloupe (diced)	9	Pineapple (diced)	15
Cantaloupe (melon)	5	Plums	17
Carrots	12	Pumpkin (canned)	10
Casaba (diced)	8	Radishes	5
Casaba (melon)	4	Raspberries (red)	17
Cauliflower	7	Sauerkraut	5
Celery	5	Squash (summer)	5
Chard	5	Squash (winter)	11
Cherries (sweet)	17	Strawberries	11
Cucumber	4	Tomatoes	6
Eggplant	6	Turnips	7
Endive	6	Watermelon (diced)	8
Grapefruit (1/2)	40	Watermelon (melon)	4
Grapes (American)	13	Zucchini	4
(European)	19		

Appendix B

THE ART OF SUBSTITUTION

Example of a daily calorie record and of substituting similar lower calorie foods for higher calorie ones. Tuesday's menu is 1274 calories lower than Monday's though the quantity of food and satisfaction it provides are quite similar.

	Monday		Tuesday	
7 am	2 scrambled eggs	222	2 poached eggs	164
	2 pcs white toast	152	2 pcs white toast	152
	1 Tbsp butter	102	2 Tbsp diet jam	40
	Coffee, 1/2 Tbsp cr		Coffee, 1/2 Tbsp non-	
	(15), 2 tsp sug (30)	45	fat milk (5), no-cal	
			sweetener(1)	6
		521		362
10 am	1 plain donut	100	1 medium orange	65
	Coffee, 1/2 Tbsp cr		Coffee, 1/2 Tbsp non-	
	(15), 2 tsp sug (30)	45	fat milk (5), no-cal	
			sweetener(1)	6
		145		71
1 pm	Swiss cheese sandwich		Swiss cheese sandwich	
	(lettuce/tomato)	300	(lettuce/tomato)	300
	1 Tbsp mayonnaise	100	1 Tbsp mustard	15
	3 choc chip cookies	150	30 grapes	90
	Coffee, 1/2 Tbsp cr		Coffee, 1/2 Tbsp non-	
	(15), 2 tsp sug (30)	45	fat milk (5), no-cal	
			sweetener(1)	6
		595		411
3 pm	1 medium apple	75	1 medium apple	75
	Coffee, 1/2 Tbsp cr		Coffee, 1/2 Tbsp non-	
	(15), 2 tsp sug (30)	45	fat milk (5), no-cal	
			sweetener(1)	6
		120		81

	Monday		Tuesday	
6 pm	1 glass white wine	100	1 glass white wine	100
	1 oz peanuts	165	4 stalks celery	28
			1 oz ricotta cheese	22
		265		150
7 pm	6 oz tomato juice	35	6 oz tomato juice	35
	small lettuce &		small lettuce &	
	tomato salad	40	tomato salad	40
	1 Tbsp 1000 Isl		1 Tbsp reduced calorie	
	Drsg	80	1000 Isl Drsg	30
	4 oz Rib Roast (lean		4 oz broiled chicken	
	with fat; weight		(no skin; weight	
	after cooking)	500	after cooking)	152
	1 baked potato	105	1 baked potato	105
	1 Tbsp butter	102	1 Tbsp sour cream	30
	1 cup green beans	35	1 cup green beans	35
		897		427
9 pm	1/2 pt strawberry		1 cup strawberries	55
	ice cream	330	3 Tbsp Cool Whip	42
	DAILY TOTAL	2873	DAILY TOTAL	1599

Appendix C

CALORIES USED IN EXERCISING

Approximate number of calories used in doing ten minutes of the following activity by a person weighing 140 pounds. Since the calorie expenditure for an activity depends on a person's weight, add 3% for each 5 pounds more, or subtract 3% for each 5 pounds less than 140 pounds that a person weighs in order to approximate greater accuracy. To adjust for a time duration other than 10 minutes, add or subtract 1/10 of the calorie expenditure for each additional or less number of minutes.

Bicycling (5 mph)	40
(10 mph)	66
Dancing rapidly	66
Fishing	39
Chopping wood (easily)	54
(rapidly)	188
Cooking	29
Digging	80
Golf	54
Ping Pong	43
Running (10 min/mile)	116
(7 min/mile)	148
Skiing (downhill)	66
(cross country-level)	91
Squash	134
Swimming	82
Tennis	70
Typing	18
Volleyball	32
Walking (level - 4 mph)	51
(uphill)	77

CALORIE GUIDE

A problem in using any calorie counting guide is to relate the size of the portion you are eating to the size of the portion described in the guide. The following guide seeks to minimize that problem by adding a second entry for each food item along with the portion size entry offered by most guides. This second entry details the calories per ounce of each food item. By knowing the calorie count for an ounce of any food, one can get a most accurate calorie count for any size portion by ascertaining the weight of the item in ounces and then multiplying by the calories per ounce for the food. To my knowledge, this is the first calorie counting guide offering calorie count information in this per-ounce format, which I believe is a real benefit to the user.

	Per Portion	Per Ounce	
Almond (in shell)	6	67	
(shelled-Tbsp)	48	170	
Anchovy	7	50	
Apple (3 to lb.)	80	16	
Apple Butter (Tbsp)	33	53	
Apple Juice (6 oz)	87	15	fl
Apple Sauce (unsweet-cup)	100	12	
(sweet-cup)	232	26	
Apricot	18	14	
(canned in syrup-cup)	222	24	
Artichoke (bud)	30	3	
Asparagus (avg. spear)	3	6	
Avocado (California)	369	37	
(Florida)	389	25	
Bacon (cooked-drained-slice 1-1/3 oz raw)	72	54	
Bamboo Shoots (cup)	41	8	
Banana (med-8-1/2″)	101	24	
Barbecue Sauce (cup)	228	26	

	Per Portion	Per Ounce
Barley (cup)	696	100
Bass (striped-oven fried-lb. raw)	896	56
Bean Sprouts (cup)	37	10
Beef (stewing-cooked-lb raw)		
(lean with fat)	994	63
(trimmed)	651	42
Beef Pot Pie (1/3 of 9″ pie)	517	70
Beer (12 oz)	151	13
Beets (cup)	54	9
Beet Greens (cup)	26	5
Biscuit (2″ diam)	103	105
Blackberries (cup)	98	13
(canned in syrup-cup)	233	25
Blueberries (cup)	90	18
Blue Fish (baked, broiled-lb-raw)	580	36
Bologna (lb)	1379	87
Boston Brown Bread (slice 3-1/4″ diam)	95	60
Bouillon (cube)	5	35
Boysenberries (cup)	88	10
Bran Flakes (40% Bran-cup)	106	85
Bread (slice)		
Cracked Wheat	66	75
French (5″ diam)	102	82
Italian	83	78
Pumpernickel	79	69
Raisin	66	74
Rye	61	69
White	76	76
Bread Crumbs (dry-cup)	392	110
Bread Pudding (with raisins-cup)	496	52
Bread Stick (4-1/4″ long)	38	110
Bread Stuffing (moist-cup)	416	59
Broccoli (med stalk)	47	7
Brussel Sprout	8	10
Bulgur (dry-cup)	602	100
(canned-cup)	230	50

	Per Portion	Per Ounce	
Butter (Tbsp)	102	203	
Whipped (Tbsp)	67	203	
Buttermilk (8 oz)	88	11	fl
Cabbage (cooked-cup)	29	6	
Cakes			
Angel Food (2-1/2″ arc-9-3/4″ diam)	161	75	
Boston Cream (2-1/8″ arc-8″ diam)	208	83	
Chocolate Devils Food (2″x2″)	143	112	
Cupcake (2-3/4″ diam)	121	100	
Fruitcake (2″x1-1/2″x1/4″)	58	110	
Gingerbread (3″x3″x2″)	371	92	
Plain cake (3″x3″x2″)	313	104	
with chocolate icing	453	105	
Pound Cake (3-1/2″x3″)	119	115	
Sponge (2-1/4″ arc-8-1/2″ diam)	131	88	
Yellow (chocolate layer 2-1/8″ arc-8″ diam)	288	100	
Candy (oz)			
Butterscotch	113	113	
Caramels	113	113	
Chocolate	144	144	
Fudge (caramel, peanut)	130	130	
(choc, van)	113	113	
Gum Drop	98	98	
Hard Candy	109	109	
Jelly Bean	104	104	
Marshmallow	90	90	
Mint (choc)	116	116	
Peanut Brittle	119	119	
Cantaloupe (melon-2 lb)	136	5	
(Diced-cup)	48	8	
Capricola (lb)	2263	141	
Carrot (7-1/2″)	30	12	
Casaba Melon (melon-4 lb)	244	4	
(Diced-cup)	46	8	
Cashews (med-1)	9	159	

	Per Portion	Per Ounce
Catsup (Tbsp)	16	30
Cauliflower (cup)	28	7
Caviar (Tbsp)	42	74
Celery (8″ stalk)	7	5
Chard (cup)	26	5
Cheeses (oz.)		
American	92	92
Blue/Roquefort	104	104
Brick	105	105
Camembert	85	85
Cheddar (domestic)	113	113
Cottage (creamed)	30	30
Cream	106	106
Limburger	98	98
Parmesan	111	111
Ricotta	22	22
Swiss	101	101
Pimiento	105	105
Process cheese spread	82	82
Cheese souffle (cup)	207	62
Cherry (sweet with pit)	5	17
(canned in syrup-cup)	208	21
Chestnut (in shell)	14	45
(shelled-cup)	310	55
Chewing Gum (piece)	5	—
Chicken (cooked-lb when raw)		
Broilers	273	18
Fryers and Roasters	570	36
Chicken a la King (cup)	468	54
Chicken Fricasse (cup)	386	46
Chicken Pot Pie (1/3 of 9″ pie)	545	68
Chickpeas (cup)	720	102
Chicory (cup)	14	5
Chili Con Carne (cup)	339	38
Chives (Tbsp)	1	—
Chocolate (bitter, baking-cup)	667	143

	Per Portion	Per Ounce
Chocolate pudding mix (4 oz pkg)	408	102
Chocolate Syrup (Tbsp)	46	92
(Fudge Syrup-Tbsp)	62	124
Chop Suey (cup)	300	34
Chow Mein (cup)	255	29
(canned-cup)	172	11
[Chuck Roast (cooked-lb raw) Chuck Steak w/ bone]		
lean w/ fat - choice	780	49
lean w/ fat - good	444	28
trimmed - choice	683	42
trimmed - good	426	26
Clam (raw-med)	8	24
Clam Nectar (6 oz)	36	6 fl
Cocoa (Tbsp)	14	75
Coconut meat (2x2)	156	98
Cod (broil with butter -lb)	771	48
Coffee (tsp)	1	37
Cookies (1)		
Brownie (chocolate icing1-1/2x1-3/4)	103	116
Butter Thin	22	130
Chocolate Chip (2-1/4" diam)	50	134
Fig Bar (1-5/8x1-5/8)	50	101
Gingersnap	29	119
Ladyfinger (3-1/4x1-3/8)	40	102
Macaroon (2-3/4" diam)	90	135
Marshmallow (choc - 1-3/4" diam)	54	116
Oatmeal (2-5/8" diam)	59	128
Peanut filled (1-3/4" diam)	58	134
Sandwich (choc. - van - 1-3/4" diam)	50	140
Sugar Wafer (3-1/2x1-1/2)	34	138
Corn (5" ear)	70	14
(canned-cup)	174	24
Corn Fritters (2" diam)	132	106
Cornbread (2-1/2x2-1/2)	161	60
Corned Beef (cooked-lb raw)	1329	83

	Per Portion	Per Ounce	
Corn Syrup (Tbsp)	59	119	fl
Crab (steamed-pieces-cup)	144	27	
Crackers (1)			
Animal	11	122	
Butter (1-7/8″ diam)	15	130	
Cheese (1-7/8″ diam)	17	136	
Graham (choc. 2-1/2″x2″x1/4″)	62	135	
(Plain 2-1/2″x2-1/2″x3/16″	28	109	
Peanut Butter Sand. (1-5/8″ sq)	35	139	
Saltines (1-7/8″ sq)	12	123	
Soda (2-3/8x2-1/8)	22	125	
Cranberries (raw-cup)	44	13	
Cranberry Juice (6 oz)	124	21	fl
Cranberry Sauce (cup)	404	42	
Cream (Tbsp)			
Half & Half	20	40	fl
Light	32	64	fl
Lt. Whipping	45	90	fl
Hvy. Whipping	53	105	fl
Cream Puff (3-1/2″ diam)	303	65	
Creamed Beef (cup)	377	44	
Cucumber (8-1/4″)	45	4	
Custard (baked-cup)	305	32	
Danish Pastry (4-1/4″ diam)	274	120	
Date (pitted)	22	77	
Deviled Ham (lb)	1592	100	
Doughnut (Pl. 3-1/2″ diam)	100	110	
Eclair (5x2)	239	68	
Eggs (large)			
Fried	99	—	
Boiled	82	—	
Poached	82	—	
Scrambled	111	—	
Eggplant (cup)	38	6	
Endive (cup)	10	6	
Farina (inst. - cup)	135	15	

	Per Portion	Per Ounce	
Fat (Tbsp)	111	250	
Fig (med)	40	23	
Fishcake (fried 3″ diam)	103	49	
(Frozen 3″ diam)	162	77	
Fish Stick (4x1)	50	50	
Flank Steak (cooked-lb raw)	596	38	
Flounder (baked with butter-lb)	916	57	
Frankfurters (5″ long - 2 oz)	176	88	
(with bun)	295	—	
Fruit cocktail (canned water pack-cup)	91	11	
(canned syrup pack-cup)	194	22	
Frozen Custard (8 oz fl)	334	42	fl
Garbanzo Beans (cup)	720	102	
Garlic (clove)	4	37	
Gelatin (cooked - cup)	142	16	
Grapefruit (3-1/2″ diam-whole)	80	5	
(sections-cup)	82	11	
Grapefruit Juice (6 oz)	78	13	fl
Grapes (American - Concord)	2	13	
(Eur. - Thom. Seedless)	3	19	
Grape Juice (6 oz)	125	21	fl
Grape Drink (6 oz)	102	17	fl
Green Beans (cup)	35	9	
Ground Beef (10% fat-cooked-lb raw)	745	47	
(21% fat-cooked-lb raw)	932	59	
Haddock (fried-lb raw)	597	37	
Ham (cooked-lb raw)	1152	72	
(trimmed)	495	31	
Hamburger (cooked - 1/4 lb raw)	233	81	
(with bun)	352	—	
Hazelnut (in shell)	9	84	
(shelled-Tbsp)	44	176	
Herring (lb plain)	943	59	
(lb-tomato sauce)	798	50	
(lb-pickled)	1012	64	
Honeydew Melon (melon-4 lb)	377	6	

	Per Portion	Per Ounce	
(diced-cup)	56	10	
Horseradish (Tbsp)	6	12	
Ice Cream (10% fat-pint)	514	33	fl
(16% fat-pint)	660	42	fl
Ice Milk (5% fat-pint)	398	25	fl
Ices (water-cup)	247	31	fl
Jams (Tbsp)	54	78	
Jellies (Tbsp)	49	77	
Kale (cup)	43	11	
Kidney Beans (cup)	220	33	
Kidney (beef - cooked - lb)	1143	71	
Knockwurst (4" - 2.4 oz)	189	79	
Kumquat (med)	12	16	
Lamb (cooked-lb raw w/ bone)			
(Leg - lean with fat)	745	47	
(Leg - trimmed)	411	26	
(Loin chops - lean with fat)	1023	101	
(Loin chops - trimmed)	368	23	
Lard (Tbsp)	117	256	
Lemon (med)	20	5	
Lemon Juice (6 oz unsweetened)	42	7	fl
Lemonade (6 oz)	81	14	fl
Lentils (cooked - cup)	212	30	
Lettuce (large leaf)	2	4	
Lima Beans (cup)	190	31	
Lime	19	7	
Lime Juice (6 oz)	48	8	fl
Limeade (6 oz)	76	13	fl
Liquor (80 proof-jigger-1-1/2 oz)	97	65	fl
(100 proof-jigger-1-1/2 oz)	124	83	fl
Liver (cooked-lb)			
Calf	1184	74	
Chicken	748	47	
Liverwurst (lb)	1393	87	
Lobster (pieces-cup)	138	27	
Lobster Newburg (cup)	485	54	

	Per Portion	Per Ounce	
Loganberries (cup)	89	18	
Loquat	6	10	
Macaroni (cooked-4 oz raw)	419	105	
Mackerel (broiled in butter- lb raw)	861	54	
Mandarin Orange (med)	39	10	
Mango	152	19	
Maple Syrup (Tbsp)	50	100	fl
Margarine (Tbsp)	102	204	
(Whipped-Tbsp)	68	204	
Marmalade (Tbsp)	51	73	
Mayonnaise (Tbsp)	100	200	
Milk (8 oz)			
Buttermilk	88	11	fl
Low Fat	145	18	fl
Low Fat-Chocolate	190	27	fl
No Fat	88	11	fl
Whole	159	20	fl
Muffins (2-5/8″ diam)			
Blueberry	112	80	
Bran	104	75	
Corn	126	90	
Mushrooms (cup)	20	8	
Mustard Greens (cup)	32	7	
Mustard (tsp)	5	28	
Nectarine	88	16	
Noodles (cooked-8 oz raw)	881	110	
Chow Mein (canned-cup)	220	139	
Oatmeal (cooked-cup)	132	16	
Oils (Tbsp)	120	240	fl
Okra (cup)	46	9	
Olive (w/ pit-med)	5	28	
Onion (raw-sliced)	44	11	
Orange (med)	65	10	
Orange juice (6 oz)	84	14	fl
Oyster (raw)	9	19	
Pancakes (4″ diam-3/8″ thick)	61	64	

	Per Portion	Per Ounce	
Papaya	119	7	
(cubed - cup)	55	11	
Parsley (cup)	26	13	
Parsnips (diced-cup)	102	19	
Peach (med)	38	10	
(canned in syrup-lb)	354	23	
Peach nectar (6 oz)	90	15	fl
Peanut (in shell)	11	111	
(shelled-Tbsp)	52	165	
Peanut butter (Tbsp)	94	167	
Pear (med)	100	17	
(syrup pack-lb)	345	22	
Pear nectar (6 oz)	96	16	fl
Peas (cup)	114	21	
(canned-cup)	164	19	
Pecan (in shell-med)	27	104	
(shelled-med)	10	195	
Pepper (sweet-lg)	36	5	
Perch (fried-lb)	1030	65	
Pickle (dill/sour-med)	7	3	
(gherkin-small)	22	40	
Pies (3-1/2" arc-9" diam)			
Apple	302	73	
Banana Custard	252	63	
Blueberry	286	70	
Cherry	308	74	
Choc. chiffon	266	90	
Cocoanut custard	268	66	
Lemon chiffon	254	87	
Lemon meringue	268	72	
Mince	320	76	
Peach	301	73	
Pecan	431	120	
Pineapple	299	73	
Pumpkin	241	60	
Rhubarb	299	73	

	Per Portion	Per Ounce
Strawberry	184	55
Pie crust mix (10 oz pkg)	1482	148
Pimientos (2 oz)	15	8
Pineapple (diced-cup)	81	15
(Syrup pack-cup)	189	21
Pineapple juice (6 oz)	112	17 fl
Pine nuts (shelled - oz)	180	180
Pistachio nuts (in shell - oz)	85	85
(shelled)	168	168
Pizza (5-1/3" arc)	155	67
Plum	7	17
(Syrup pack-cup)	214	23
Pomegranate	97	10
Popcorn (popped-plain-cup)	23	108
(popped-oil & salt-cup)	41	127
Pork (loin & loin chops-cooked lb raw-no bone)	1115	70
Porterhouse steak (cooked - lb raw)		
(lean w/ fat)	1400	88
(trimmed)	385	25
Potatoes		
(baked in skin-med)	105	21
(boiled in skin-med)	104	20
(French fried-10 med)	137	78
(hash brown-cup)	355	65
(mashed-cup)	197	27
Potato chip (1-3/4"x2-1/2")	12	161
Pretzels (3" long x 1/2" diam)	20	111
Prunes (cooked-cup)	504	51
Prune juice (6 oz)	148	25 fl
Pumpkin (canned-cup)	81	10
(seeds-cup)	774	157
Rabbit (stewed-lb raw)	529	33
Radishes (cup)	20	5
Raisins (Tbsp)	26	82
Raspberries (black-cup)	98	21

	Per Portion	Per Ounce
(red-cup)	70	17
Rhubarb (raw-cup)	20	4
Rib roast (cooked-lb raw w/ bone)		
(lean w/ fat)	1342	84
(trimmed)	470	30
Rice (cooked-brown-cup)	232	34
(cooked-white-cup)	223	31
Rockfish (steamed-lb raw)	396	25
Rolls		
Cloverleaf (2-1/2″ diam)	83	83
Frankfurter	119	85
Hamburger	119	85
Hard roll (3-3/4″ diam)	156	88
Rolls from mix (2-1/2″ diam)	105	85
Round steak (cooked-lb raw-w/ bone)		
(lean w/ fat)	793	50
(trimmed)	491	31
Salad dressing (Tbsp)		
Blue/Roquefort	76	145
French	66	115
Italian	83	160
Mayonnaise	100	200
Russian	74	140
Thousand Island	80	140
Salami (lb)	2041	128
Salmon (broiled, baked fillet-lb)	826	52
Salmon (canned-lb)		
Atlantic, Chinook	938	58
Chum, pink	640	40
Coho	694	44
Sardines (canned in oil-lb)	1411	88
(drained-lb)	921	58
Sauerkraut (cup)	42	5
Sausage (cooked-patty 2 oz raw)	129	65
(cooked link-1 oz raw)	62	62
Scallops (steamed-lb)	508	32

	Per Portion	Per Ounce
Sesame seeds (Tbsp)	47	163
Shad (baked-lb-raw fillets)	734	46
Sherbet (orange-pt)	516	33 fl
Shrimp (fried - lb)	1021	64
(canned - lb)	526	33
Sirloin steak (cooked-lb raw)		
(lean w/ fat)	1192	75
(trimmed)	420	27
Sodas (12 oz)		
Colas, Cream, Root Beer	150	13
Fruit flavored	171	15
Ginger Ale, Quinine	113	10
Soups (canned, condensed, water added-cup)		
Asparagus, cream of	65	8
Bean w/ pork	168	19
Beef bouillon	31	4
Beef noodle	67	8
Chicken consomme	22	3
Chicken, cream of	94	11
Chicken gumbo	55	7
Chicken w/ rice	48	6
Clam chowder (Man.)	81	10
Minestrone	105	13
Mushroom	134	16
Onion	65	8
Pea	130	15
Tomato	88	10
Turkey noodle	79	9
Vegetable	78	9
Sour Cream (Tbsp)	30	60
Soy sauce (Tbsp)	12	25
Spaghetti (cooked-cup)	192	42
Spare ribs (cooked-lb raw)	792	50
Spinach (cup)	41	7
Squash (summer-cup)	25	5

	Per Portion	Per Ounce	
(winter-cup)	93	11	
Strawberries (fresh-cup)	55	11	
(frozen-cup)	278	31	
Sturgeon (smoked-lb)	676	42	
Sugar (granulated-tsp)	15	105	
(lump)	19	105	
(powdered-tsp)	10	105	
Sunflower seeds (shelled - oz)	159	159	
Sweetbreads (calf, lamb-lb)	730	48	
(beef-lb)	1450	90	
Sweet potatoes (baked-5″)	161	32	
(candied-pc 2-1/2″x2″ precook)	143	48	
Swordfish (cooked-lb raw)	499	32	
T-bone steak (cooked-lb raw)			
lean w/ fat	1395	88	
trimmed	368	23	
Tangerine (med)	39	9	
Tapioca pudding (cup)	221	37	
Tartar sauce (Tbsp)	74	148	
Tomato (med)	20	6	
Tomato juice (6 oz)	35	6	fl
Tomato paste (cup)	215	24	
Tongue (beef-cooked-lb)	1107	70	
Tuna fish (canned-oil-lb)	1306	82	
drained	894	56	
in water	576	36	
Turkey (no skin-lb)			
(light meat)	798	50	
(dark meat)	921	58	
Turkey pot pie (1/3 of 9″ pie)	550	67	
Turnips (cup)	36	7	
Veal (boneless stew-cooked-lb raw)	703	44	
Vegetable juice (6 oz)	30	5	fl
Vinegar (Tbsp)	2	4	fl
Waffle (7″ diam x 5/8″ thick)	206	78	
Walnut (Black-in shell-oz)	40	40	

	Per Portion	Per Ounce	
(shelled-Tbsp)	50	178	
(Persian or English-in shell-oz)	83	83	
(shelled-Tbsp)	52	185	
Waterchestnut	12	18	
Watercress (cup)	7	5	
Watermelon (slice 10″ diam x 1″ thick)	111	4	
(Diced pieces-cup)	42	8	
Wax/yellow beans (cup)	28	7	
Wheat germ (Tbsp)	23	108	
White fish (smoked-lb)	703	44	
(baked, stuffed-lb)	976	61	
Wine (table-12% alcohol-4 oz)	100	25	fl
(dessert-18% alcohol-2 oz)	81	41	fl
Yogurt (whole milk-cup)	152	19	
Zucchini (cup)	22	4	

Aids in Remembering

As I have said repeatedly throughout this book, we must keep the ideas alive in our memory and we must arouse and refresh our energy. A valuable assist in helping one to remember comes from hearing the right message on a cassette tape as well as seeing it on the printed page. You gain power from repeatedly hearing the right voice giving the right message. It arouses the energy. It brings the ideas to life. I have prepared each of the following 60-minute cassette tapes to be inspirational as well as instructive. They will help you keep the message in mind and stimulate your thinking the right thing at the right moment. They will inspire you to act. Play them repeatedly and they will keep your mind set in the direction of weight control; and they will keep your energy aroused.

GETTING STARTED   This tape is designed to get you started on your weight control program; to stop procrastinating; to stop waiting until next Monday.

MID-STREAM   This tape is designed to keep you going once you have started, until you have reached your goal; to not let up as all failed dieters do.

KEEPING IT OFF	This tape is designed to make sure you do not gain any of the weight back once you have reached your goal.
INTENTION MAKES IT HAPPEN	Intention is the magical ingredient that makes things happen effortlessly. This tape tells you what intention is and how to create it.

Individual tapes are $10.00. The complete set of four is $30.00—a 25% discount. If you are not satisfied, you may return the tapes within ten days of receiving them for a full refund.

Order by sending your name and mailing address along with payment by check, money order or VISA or MASTER-CARD to Jon Perlow, P.O. Box 616, Mill Valley, California, 94941. California residents add 6% sales tax. If paying by credit card, please indicate whether Visa Or Mastercard, the card number, the date of expiration and the exact name of the cardholder as it appears on the card.